Praise for *Build* of *Ownership in Healthcare*

"Culture is everything. It will make or break your organization. In this book, authors Joe Tye and Bob Dent offer us an easy, step-by-step process to instill a culture of excellence. I am confident that this book can assist health-care leaders in building a culture of ownership to ensure that we stage the best possible experience for people in need of healthcare services."

–Sylvain Trepanier, DNP, RN, CENP
System Chief Nursing Officer
Premier Health

"Tye and Dent give us insightful views into the underpinnings of culture and offer a blueprint for leaders within and beyond healthcare for significant and successful change."

–Michelle A. Janney, PhD, RN, NEA-BC, FAAN
Executive Vice President and Chief Nurse Executive
Indiana University Health
Associate Dean for Clinical Affairs
Indiana University School of Nursing

"Joe Tye and Bob Dent have captured the essence of what makes truly great organizations—shared values and a culture that engages everyone. Their messages are timely, practical, and incredibly useful. Their ideas will inspire, engage, and create remarkable results in any business environment. I highly recommend that every leader take the time to read this important book."

–Nancy M. Schlichting
Retired CEO, Henry Ford Health System
Chairperson, Commission on Care
Director, Walgreens Boots Alliance and Hill-Rom Holdings Inc.

"These two authors have created a magnificent work of both practical and transformational knowledge in leadership with the 'how to' that so often is missing from books on leadership. Their approach to culture building makes clear the importance of aligning values with not only words, but actions that leaders must deliver with authenticity and presence. The analogy with architecture and infrastructure is visually brilliant, as we are building cultures to stand the test of time and weather the elements of unpredictability and complexity."

–Cole Edmonson, DNP, RN, FACHE, NEA-BC, FAAN
Chief Nursing Officer
Texas Health Presbyterian Hospital, Dallas

"In these challenging times, healthcare organizations struggle to increase patient and employee satisfaction, along with fiscal stability. The solution lies in Building a Culture of Ownership in Healthcare. *The proven strategies outlined by Bob Dent and Joe Tye equip healthcare professionals with the inspiration, purpose, and specific tools to improve the emotional climate and culture in the workplace, where employees are positive, self-empowered, and fully engaged. Rarely has a book so brilliantly combined science and humanity with stories, chapter summaries, and questions for individual application and success. Investing in this book is an investment in your organization, your people—and your highest quality of patient care."*

–LeAnn Thieman, LPN, CSP, CPAE
Author, *Chicken Soup for the Nurse's Soul* series &
SelfCare for HealthCare™

"A variety of healthcare leaders have identified organizational culture as a major factor underlying patient care quality and workforce engagement challenges. Joe Tye and Bob Dent believe that nurse leaders can take specific actions to change culture for the better. This practical, straightforward, and story-filled book should serve as a guide for nurse leaders who want to create an environment of ownership where both patients and staff will thrive."

–Kathleen Sanford, DBA, RN, FACHE, FAAN
Senior VP and CNO, Catholic Health Initiatives
Editor-In Chief, *Nursing Administration Quarterly*

"Finally, a book that describes how we can change culture at any level! It is vital for nursing leaders to understand their invisible architecture so they can create positive change. This book provides must-read information that all nurses need to create a culture that supports employees and patients."

–Jennifer Mensik, PhD, RN, NEA-BC, FAAN
Executive Director, Nursing, Medicine and
Pharmacy Programs at OnCourse Learning
Instructor, Arizona State University DNP program

"Tye and Dent have written a tour de force. The book is chock-full of compelling ideas, actionable advice, meaningful stories, and proven strategies. It is the best treatment of the challenging topic of organizational culture that I have read. This is not a book to skim as there are delectable insights on every page. Read every word and put into action their spot-on advice about achieving cultures of ownership."

–David Altman, PhD
Chief Operating Officer
Center for Creative Leadership

BUILDING A CULTURE OF OWNERSHIP IN HEALTHCARE

The Invisible Architecture of Core Values, Attitude, and Self-Empowerment

Joe Tye, MHA, MBA

Bob Dent, DNP, MBA, RN, NEA-BC, CENP, FACHE

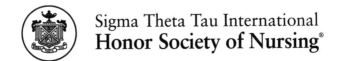

Sigma Theta Tau International
Honor Society of Nursing®

The Honor Society of Nursing, Sigma Theta Tau International (STTI) is a nonprofit organization founded in 1922 whose mission is advancing world health and celebrating nursing excellence in scholarship, leadership, and service. Members include practicing nurses, instructors, researchers, policymakers, entrepreneurs, and others. STTI has more than 500 chapters located at more than 700 institutions of higher education throughout Armenia, Australia, Botswana, Brazil, Canada, Colombia, England, Ghana, Hong Kong, Japan, Kenya, Lebanon, Malawi, Mexico, the Netherlands, Pakistan, Portugal, Singapore, South Africa, South Korea, Swaziland, Sweden, Taiwan, Tanzania, Thailand, the United Kingdom, and the United States of America. More information about STTI can be found online at www.nursingsociety.org.

Sigma Theta Tau International
550 West North Street
Indianapolis, IN, USA 46202

To order additional books, buy in bulk, or order for corporate use, contact Nursing Knowledge International at 888.NKI.4YOU (888.654.4968/US and Canada) or +1.317.634.8171 (outside US and Canada).

To request a review copy for course adoption, email solutions@nursingknowledge.org or call 888. NKI.4YOU (888.654.4968/US and Canada) or +1.317.634.8171 (outside US and Canada).

To request author information, or for speaker or other media requests, contact Marketing, Honor Society of Nursing, Sigma Theta Tau International at 888.634.7575 (US and Canada) or +1.317.634.8171 (outside US and Canada).

ISBN:	9781945157172
EPUB ISBN:	9781945157189
PDF ISBN:	9781945157196
MOBI ISBN:	9781945157202

Library of Congress Cataloging-in-Publication Data

Names: Tye, Joe, 1951- author. | Dent, Bob, 1966- author. | Tye, Doug, author.

Title: Building a culture of ownership in healthcare : the invisible architecture of core values, attitude, and self-empowerment / Joe Tye, Bob Dent, Doug Tye.

Description: Indianapolis, IN : Sigma Theta Tau International, 2017. | Includes bibliographical references.

Identifiers: LCCN 2017002653 (print) | LCCN 2017004016 (ebook) | ISBN 9781945157172 (print : alk. paper) | ISBN 9781945157189 (EPUB) | ISBN 9781945157196 (PDF) | ISBN 9781945157202 (MOBI) | ISBN 9781945157189 (Epub) | ISBN 9781945157196 (Pdf) | ISBN 9781945157202 (Mobi)

Subjects: | MESH: Delivery of Health Care--organization & administration | Organizational Culture | Attitude of Health Personnel | Leadership

Classification: LCC RA418 (print) | LCC RA418 (ebook) | NLM W 84.1 | DDC 362.1--dc23

LC record available at https://lccn.loc.gov/2017002653

Second Printing, 2018

Publisher: Dustin Sullivan

Acquisitions Editor: Emily Hatch

Editorial Coordinator: Paula Jeffers

Cover Design: TnT Design, Inc.

Interior Design & Composition: TnT Design, Inc.

Indexer: Larry Sweazy

Principal Book Editor: Carla Hall

Development Editor: Rebecca Senninger

Project Editor: Rebecca Senninger

Copy Editor: Rebecca Whitney

Proofreader: Todd Lothery

Dedications

Joe dedicates this book with love and pride to Doug Tye, PhD—we could not have done it without you!

Bob dedicates this book to his family: grandmother, Helen Fuller Logsdon; father, Bob Goforth; stepfather, Howard Dent; and mother, Janice Dent, for raising four boys, including Mark, Mike, and Lee, who all became men in nursing.

Acknowledgments

From both of us:

This book would not have been possible without a host of people we're honored to consider part of an invisible architecture that supports a culture of ownership. First, at the heart of the work we do, but more importantly friends, are Michelle Arduser and Kim Kincaid. They have assisted each of us as we have taken time to work, research, and write.

We are grateful to those who gave of their time and talents in interviews or contributed stories to be included in this work. We especially appreciate the generous contributions of Bonnie and Mark Barnes and Tim Porter-O'Grady. More than 100 people participated in interviews or submitted stories, some of which we will need to save for the next book. Rather than run the risk of leaving anyone out, we simply say thank you to everyone who shared their stories with us.

A special thank you to the tremendous team at Sigma Theta Tau International. This book was born the day STTI's acquiring book editor, Emily Hatch, approached us after our presentation at the annual AONE conference and said, "You guys should write a book." Carla Hall was our principal book editor, Rebecca Senninger was our development editor, and Rebecca Whitney was our copy editor. They made the process easy, enjoyable, and (relatively) painless.

From Joe:

I wish I could individually acknowledge all of the leaders (formal and informal) we have worked with at Values Coach, but I will single out several to whom I owe a particular debt of gratitude for their support of our work—special appreciation for these people and their teams: Patrick Charmel (CEO of Griffin Hospital), Todd Linden (CEO of Grinnell Regional Medical Center), Judy Rich (CEO of Tucson Medical Center), Ryan Smith (CEO of Memorial Hospital of Converse County), Charlie Button (CEO of Star Valley Medical Center), Paul Utemark (CEO of Fillmore County Hospital), Nancy Howell Agee (CEO of Carilion Clinic), Ed Lamb (CEO of Mount Carmel Health System), Deb Wilson (COO of Kalispell Regional Healthcare), Susan Hall (director of organizational development at Guthrie Clinic), Lamont Yoder (CEO of Banner Gateway Medical Center/MD Anderson Cancer Center), Brad Neet (CEO of Southwest Healthcare System), Carol Wahl (CNO at CHI Good

Samaritan Hospital), Bakhita Al-Khabbash (manager for organizational learning, Sidra Medical and Research Center in Qatar), Jeff Harrold (chairman and CEO of Auto-Owners Insurance Company), Susan Frampton (president of Planetree), Laura Redoutey (president of the Nebraska Hospital Association), Jerry Jurena (president of the North Dakota Hospital Association), Elisa White (vice president at the Arkansas Hospital Association), Martha Harrell (vice president at the Georgia Hospital Association), and many, many more names that I would add if I could. Above all, I want to acknowledge the team at Midland Health—especially CEO Russell Meyers, COO/CNO Bob Dent, vice president of planning and marketing Marcy Madrid, Master Certified Values Coach Trainer Alisha Acosta, and the team of 60 Certified Values Coach Trainers.

The Values Coach Advisory Board provides me with essential guidance and encouragement, and I want to acknowledge members Tony Burke, Bob Dent, Sandra Fancher, Traci Fenton, Sam Houston, Todd Linden, and Jim Seifert. Dave Altman, chief operating officer at the Center for Creative Leadership, has been a friend, an advisor, and a co-conspirator for more than three decades. Friend and author Steve Pressfield has encouraged me in my writing in more ways than he will ever know, and Gary Ryan Blair challenges me to remember that everything counts.

The Veterans Health Administration has received considerable criticism in recent years, some of which is recounted in this book, but I want to acknowledge my respect and admiration for the people who serve our veterans, and for the leaders who opened doors for Values Coach, including Alex Spector, Susan Pendergrass, Michael Fisher, Vic Rosenbaum, and Ken Kizer. I appreciate Kris Lukish, vice president of human resources at HCA West Florida, for introducing me to the division's HR team and guiding me to background resources about HCA.

I also want to acknowledge the Vietnam crew, including Thuy Do, our former CFO who created the template for our webinar programs; Hung Viet Tran, who has grown the little business he started in a Values Coach cubicle into GotIt!—one of the hottest companies in Silicon Valley and Vietnam; Tung Hoang, who has progressed from shooting Values Coach videos to becoming CEO of iflix Vietnam; and, above all, my dear friend Kien Pham, the most courageous man I know, who has transformed from Vietnam boat refugee to one of the most respected business leaders and philanthropists in both of the countries that he can now call home.

Finally, I want to thank my family. Happiness is being married to your best friend, and my best friend, Sally, also happens to work in the Values Coach office, so I am truly blessed. Annie, with her brand-new PhD in neurosciences from the University of Iowa, has set her sights on promoting scientific knowledge in the world of public policy. Doug, with his brand-new PhD in American literature from Johns Hopkins University, was a full partner with Bob and me in the creation of this book. Michelle Arduser is the director of client services at Values Coach, but I include her here because, to me, she is more family than she is coworker.

From Bob:

I would like to personally thank Donna Boatright for starting a medical explorers' program in the 1980s that launched me into my nursing career. I would like to recognize Rhonda Anderson as a professional soulmate for mentoring me as I became a nurse leader. Thanks to those at the American Organization of Nurse Executives (AONE), the voice of nursing leadership: Pamela Thompson, Maureen Swick, and the staff. I also want to thank those I had the opportunity to serve with on the AONE board of directors and on the Texas Organization of Nurse Executives board of directors. I would like to acknowledge and thank the faculty and staff at Texas Tech University Health Sciences Center School of Nursing (especially Barbara Cherry, Alexia Green, and Patricia Yoder-Wise). I would also like to acknowledge my friends and colleagues with the American Nurses Association, Texas Nurses Association, Sigma Theta Tau International, and the Iota Mu chapter. A special thanks to my friends and coworkers at Midland Memorial Hospital, who have woven the culture of ownership into the DNA of the organization and who are making a real difference every day—especially Russell Meyers, Marcy Madrid, Alisha Acosta, Sari Nabulsi, Lawrence Wilson, Kim Kincaid, and the 60 Midland Health Certified Values Coach Trainers. Without their belief and their desire to create a great place to work and an excellent patient care experience, this book would never have happened.

And lastly, a profound thanks and appreciation to my wife, Karen, for being there for me throughout my career. She has been my inspiration and motivation every step of the way. She has sacrificed so much in support of my career and our family. I also thank my wonderful children, whom I love and adore: Adam and his wife, Jackie; Joshua and his wife, Diana, and their two beautiful daughters, Adaline and Ella; Timothy; Abigail; and Rachel.

About the Authors

Joe Tye, MHA, MBA, is the CEO and head coach of Values Coach Inc., which provides consulting, training, and coaching on values-based leadership and cultural transformation for hospital, corporate, and association clients. He founded Values Coach in 1994 with the purpose of "transforming people through the power of values and transforming organizations through the power of people."

Joe earned a master's degree in hospital administration from the University of Iowa and an MBA from the Stanford Graduate School of Business, where he was class co-president. He is the author or coauthor of 15 books* and more than 100 articles, webinars, and video programs on personal achievement, effective leadership, and organizational culture. He created the course The Twelve Core Action Values, which is often referred to this way: "like graduate school for the seven habits." At Values Coach, Joe and his team use the tools and techniques described in this book to help healthcare organizations build a stronger and more vibrant culture of ownership on a foundation of values.

Before founding Values Coach, Joe was chief operating officer for a large community teaching hospital. On the volunteer front, he was the founding president of the Association of Air Medical Services and a leading activist fighting against unethical tobacco industry marketing practices; his work to fight white-collar drug pushers was profiled in the Pulitzer Prize–winning book *Ashes to Ashes*. Joe and his wife, Sally, who have two adult children, live on a small farmstead in Iowa; their second home is a tent in the Grand Canyon.

---

*Joe and Bob have written two other books together: *The Heart of a Nurse Leader: Values-Based Leadership for Healthcare Organizations* and *Pickle Pledge: Creating a More Positive Healthcare Culture – One Attitude at a Time*. Joe is also author of *The Florence Prescription: From Accountability to Ownership*, *All Hands on Deck: 8 Essential Lessons for Building a Culture of Ownership*, and a dozen other books that are available through online retailers.

Bob Dent, DNP, MBA, RN, NEA-BC, CENP, FACHE, is the senior vice president, chief operating, and chief nursing officer at Midland Memorial Hospital in Midland, Texas, and the 2018 President of the American Organization of Nurse Executives (AONE). He maintains academic appointments with Texas Tech University Health Sciences Center School of Nursing and the University of Texas of the Permian Basin. He is the recipient of the 2016 Richard Hader Visionary Leader Award by *Nursing Management*; the 2014 Distinguished Alumni Award by Texas Tech University Health Sciences Center School of Nursing; the Excellence in Leadership Award by the Texas Organization of Nurse Executives in 2013; the Nursing Excellence Award for Transformational Leadership by his colleagues at Midland Memorial Hospital in 2011; the Healthcare Leadership Award by Clairvia in 2010; and the Class of 2006 Up and Comer of the Year by *Modern Healthcare* magazine.

With 30 years of diverse experience in healthcare, Bob has served as a nursing assistant, licensed vocational nurse, registered nurse, licensed nursing home administrator, chief nursing officer, and chief operating officer of small and large organizations. He has also served as dean of the health sciences center of a local community college. A community college graduate, Bob's first degree was an associate of applied science. He went on to earn a bachelor of science in nursing, a master of business administration/healthcare management, and, finally, a doctorate of nursing practice (DNP) from Texas Tech University Health Sciences Center School of Nursing.

Bob is active in many professional nursing organizations and has served on multiple boards over the years. He now serves on the boards of Midland YMCA, Hospice of Midland, the Texas Tech University Health Sciences Center alumni association, Values Coach Inc., Texas Hospital Associations HOSPAC, and the University of Phoenix Center for Healthcare Research International executive advisory board. He and his wife of more than 27 years have five children and two grandchildren. Before joining Midland Memorial Hospital in 2007, Bob was the associate administrator and chief nursing officer of Banner Health's Sterling Regional MedCenter in Sterling, Colorado.

Table of Contents

Introduction

Joe's first visit to Midland, Texas, was in May of 2012 for a nursing leadership retreat at Midland Memorial Hospital (MMH), where Bob works. MMH was constructing a new $176 million hospital tower. The day after the retreat, Bob and Joe donned hard hats for a tour. Bob's pride and excitement were obvious during the tour. The new building was needed to replace facilities that had been constructed not long after the end of the Second World War. That need was made more urgent by unacceptably low patient satisfaction scores. The new tower, it was expected, would remedy that problem.

The new facility opened at the end of 2012, and it was indeed beautiful, having been designed with patients, families, and staff members in mind. Private patient rooms feature an expansive view of West Texas, while ceiling-mounted automatic patient lifts over every single bed ensure that no nurse would ever suffer a back injury while trying to lift a patient. (MMH was one of the first in the nation to make this commitment.) A full-service cafeteria offers a wide range of gourmet and healthful food options, and on sunny days people can sit outside in a courtyard that features a walking labyrinth. From the nurses' station to the chapel, every detail was designed to make the new facility beautiful and functional.

Despite the aesthetic beauty and operational ease, though, patient satisfaction failed to go up. Unfortunately, it actually continued to fall after the new facility opened. By the end of 2013, patient satisfaction scores were at record low levels. The accrediting agency cited the organization's leadership for not having appropriately addressed these scores. Worse yet, there was mounting evidence that employee disengagement was on the rise. These problems weren't reflected only in patient satisfaction survey scores; they were increasingly obvious from the tone of patient letters, coverage by the local media, and staff conversations in hallways and break rooms.

At that point, Bob remembered Joe's presentation about the "Invisible Architecture" of an organization, a construction metaphor in which the foundation is core values, the superstructure is organizational culture, and the interior finish is workplace attitude. Joe called this "the blueprint behind the blueprint." To the MMH leadership team, it was increasingly clear that in opening the new building, they had raised patient expectations, but in not simultaneously working on the Invisible Architecture, they had actually increased the gap between higher expectations and actual experience.

Over the succeeding 3 years, Values Coach has partnered with the team at MMH to implement many of the strategies described in this book. The initiative was launched during Nurses Week and Hospital Week of 2014 with every employee being given a copy of Joe's book, *The Florence Prescription: From Accountability to Ownership*, with a special foreword by four senior members of the MMH executive team. Results of the first Culture Assessment Survey (CAS), which were not a source of pride, were shared with everyone along with a challenge to do better. MMH was the first hospital in the nation to commit to The Pickle Pledge and to undertake The Pickle Challenge for Charity*. During a 1-week period, the hospital turned more than 4,000 individual episodes of complaining into 25-cent contributions to the hospital's emergency employee catastrophic assistance fund.

People at every level of the organization were engaged in a dialogue about the values at MMH; a new statement of values was defined and innovatively presented in Joe's new book, *Pioneer Spirit, Caring Heart, Healing Mission*—featuring a story that built on the history and traditions of the organization and the community—that was given to every employee. Appreciating the importance of connecting personal and organizational values, more than 60 MMH employees have become Certified Values Coach Trainers (CVCT) and now teach the 60-module course on The Twelve Core Action Values in a 2-day format that all current and new employees must complete.

---

*The Pickle Pledge is a promise that one makes to oneself and to one's team that they will turn complaints and frustrations into blessings and/or constructive suggestions. It is a promise to help create and sustain a more positive environment that is free from bullying, disrespect, and other forms of toxic emotional negativity. The Pickle Challenge for Charity is a 1-week period during which people who complain deposit a quarter, or are invited by a coworker to deposit a quarter, into a decorated pickle jar with all proceeds being donated to a charity chosen by the organization. The Pickle Pledge is described in Chapter 7. You can read more in the 2016 book, *Pickle Pledge: Creating a More Positive Healthcare Culture—One Attitude at a Time*, by Joe Tye and Bob Dent.

MMH now has a Culture of Ownership training room and a Culture of Ownership page on the hospital's website. Immediately outside the training room, a large framed poster says "Proceed Until Apprehended: Leadership Does Not Require a Management Title" (a line from *The Florence Prescription*), which is a philosophy the leadership team has worked hard to promote. Every morning at 8:16 sharp, leaders and anyone else who wishes to participate (including patients and visitors) join in the Daily Leadership Huddle in the main lobby to reaffirm MMH's commitment to being emotionally positive, self-empowered, and fully engaged, and to hear an update about hospital operations. During the day, the same information is shared in huddles across the organization.

The results have been remarkable. In many areas of the hospital, patient satisfaction has gone from record-low (1st percentile) to record-high (90th percentile in the emergency department with significant improvements with inpatient satisfaction as well), and there has been a 180-degree shift in the tenor of letters received from patients and in media coverage. Employee engagement is the best it has ever been, which is reflected in best-ever clinical quality outcomes and determinants of value-based purchasing. For example, MMH has experienced a 68% reduction in clostridium difficile infections, a 50% reduction in central-line associated blood stream infections, and a 38% reduction in ventilator-related events. As of this writing, MMH has gone 180 days without a significant event being reported in the Daily Leadership Huddle. Nursing turnover has decreased 32%, with a 43% reduction in turnover of nurses hired since we began our Culture of Ownership at MMH. Joe estimated the annual cultural productivity benefit to be more than $7 million, which MMH leadership considers to be an underestimate. While everyone loves the beautiful new building, an investment in the Invisible Architecture within that building of well under one-half of 1% of the cost of the visible architecture has probably had a bigger impact on employee engagement, patient satisfaction, and community reputation.

The best part is the impact that the Culture of Ownership initiative has had on the lives of the people who have embraced it. We share several of their stories in this book, as well as stories from those at other organizations embracing a culture of ownership.

The book itself is organized in three parts. Part 1 (Chapters 1 and 2) describes the Invisible Architecture model and the importance of building a culture of ownership, illustrated with examples of values statements, culture codes, and attitude expectations (both best and worst) from healthcare and other industries. Part 2 (Chapters 3-5) further describes elements of the Invisible Architecture model in which the foundation is core values, the superstructure is organizational culture, and the interior finish is workplace attitude. Part 3 (Chapters 6-10) covers the importance of values-based leadership for fostering and sustaining a culture of ownership. Throughout this book, we will share examples from real-world organizations, including many from industries outside healthcare (where the most progressive culture practices are often pioneered). Our focus in this book is on healthcare culture in particular, but healthcare organizations can learn and grow by paying attention to 'what works—and what doesn't work—in other fields.

Finally, a key message in this book is that culture does not change unless and until people change, and people will not change unless they are given tools and structure and become inspired to make the commitment to use them.

Building a culture of ownership at MMH has been more than a gift to those who work there. It has also been an investment in the organization and the community. We hope it will be for you as well.

Joe Tye and Bob Dent

Foreword

RADCRAP with Faith. That's the mnemonic device we use to remember the sequence of The Self Empowerment Pledge promises. Responsibility, Accountability, Determination, Contribution, Resilience, And Perspective; with Faith. When Joe Tye first gave us a set of his multicolored bracelets, one for each promise, we could immediately see the power behind this simple concept of reciting a promise each day that would impact the way we look at our lives and how we interact with others. Our favorite promise is Perspective, and not just because it is Saturday's Promise. It reads: "Though I might not understand why adversity happens, by my conscious choice I will find strength, compassion, and grace through my trials." We wear a lavender Perspective bracelet every day. Why?

In late 1999, our son Patrick (Pat)—33 years old, a brand-new father to baby girl Riley, and a most loving husband to his wife, Tena—died of complications from the autoimmune disease nicknamed ITP. With Pat hospitalized for 8 weeks, we were exposed for the first time to our healthcare system when it deals with the most critically ill people and their families. Without going into the details of those worst weeks of our lives, suffice it to say that when Pat died, we as a family needed to find something to turn our attention to that was not life-threatening, gruesome, negative, or painful. While we knew that nothing would help us make sense of Pat's untimely death, we had to find something to fill the gaping hole in our hearts that losing him had left. We had to find something positive. And we found it in our memories of the numerous nurses who cared for him during those 8 weeks.

As a family, we expected that when a loved one is in a good hospital, the care will be competent. True to form, Pat's nurses were clinically excellent. What we did not expect, and what really got our attention, were the compassion, kindness, and sensitivity his nurses showed to Pat, even when he was totally sedated, and that his nurses showed to us, even when we were family members hovering over a loved one, asking the same questions again and again, fearing for the life of our Patrick, and surely not at our best. When Pat died, we were filled with gratitude to those nurses. We expected that the nurses at Pat's bedside were not unique. Nurses around the world demonstrate those same qualities every day in the huge lifesaving effort they make and in the little actions they perform that make a great difference in a patient's and family's experience.

We had to say thank you to nurses, so we created The DAISY Award for Extraordinary Nurses. DAISY stands for Diseases Attacking the Immune System, since Pat had one. Our goal was to provide a means for patients, families, and colleagues to express their gratitude by sharing and celebrating in a meaningful way the stories of their extraordinary nurses. Little did we know when we started DAISY that there was no recognition program honoring what nurses become nurses to do—care for people. So the impact of The DAISY Award and the support by nurse leaders and organizations were tremendous. As of this writing, The DAISY Award is celebrating nurses in over 2,300 healthcare facilities in all 50 United States and internationally. Nearly a million nominations have been written so far. Clearly, we are not the only people who want to say thank you to their nurses!

One of the hospitals that adopted our program was Midland Memorial Hospital in Texas. Chief nursing officer (and now also chief operating officer) Bob Dent explained to us that The DAISY Award was a perfect fit for the positive environment he was building for patients and his workforce. We knew that the stories DAISY solicits focus on all the "right" going on in healthcare. What we did not appreciate was the cultural impact this focus would have. Bob was among many prominent nurse executives who helped us understand that while we were using the powerful expression of gratitude to cope with our grief, nurse leaders and organizations were using that gratitude to help create a positive work environment where the patient experience and employee satisfaction would benefit.

Bob insisted we get to know Joe Tye and learn about his construct for Invisible Architecture. Joe's goals for the organizations he works with and DAISY's are well-aligned. His core values lead to a positive workplace attitude that is more efficient and effective for patient care. DAISY celebrates the actions that take place in that positive workplace with the knowledge that what is celebrated provides outstanding role models for all, taking an organization's mission/vision/values statements off the hospital wall and bringing them to life in day-to-day care.

Joe describes how to create a culture in which employees not only take ownership for their work but also hold their patients and families to their hearts and do their very best for them because it's the right thing to do. DAISY Award Honorees own their practices and their relationships with patients and families. They are proud of the work they do yet oh-so-humbled when it is recognized. "I didn't do anything special. I was just doing my job" is the most frequent response by nurses when it is announced that they are being honored. Taking ownership for their care is, to these "DAISY Nurses," ordinary. But to those of us on the receiving end of that care, it is extraordinary, and we celebrate those special nurses who provide it. Invisible Architecture creates the space for this extraordinary care to live and breathe, impacting patient care quality and experience.

Understanding the principles of Invisible Architecture has helped us as co-CEOs and full-time volunteers of The DAISY Foundation to understand the culture our own organization has built. There are now nearly 20 people working at DAISY. We work out of our homes in Annapolis, Atlanta, Detroit, Northern California, Oklahoma City, and Seattle. Only our executive director is a nurse, and the rest of us have experienced the impact nurses have on us as patients and families. We connect with each other thanks to an online database we share, an online meeting resource, online shared files, and telephones. Most importantly, we are connected by a commitment to our shared mission that we never lose sight of—our passion to say thank you to nurses for their extraordinary care and compassion.

Everyone on our staff owns her or his work. John, who ships out DAISY Award gifts, packs with loving care and answers every email from a hospital with an uplifting quote or a photo that makes the reader smile or laugh. Every Friday, Janet sends "good news" emails to ensure that we head into the weekend knowing the impact DAISY has made that week. Christina works on her laptop as she recovers from spine surgery, not wanting to miss a request from a hospital looking for information about DAISY or the opportunity to help one of our current partners make their program even better with a best-practices webinar. Peter and Jennifer tend to the details of our finances with such attention to detail that you would think it was their money, not DAISY's. Cindy S manages a significant load of abstract, article, and presentation writing, ensuring that DAISY has a presence and a voice in the nursing profession in ways we cannot achieve without her expertise and insight as a nurse. Cindy L, our *pro bono* researcher, is relentless in researching the impact of our program, helping us understand how The DAISY Award is making a difference. Melissa and Tena, our beloved daughters-in-law, have both experienced firsthand the best of nursing. They—along with Amy, Dana, Julie, Kara, and Lisa—work tirelessly to ensure that our gratitude is felt and that implementing The DAISY Award is a creative and rewarding process for the nurses who run it at their hospitals. Dianne reads every DAISY Honoree story that is registered with us, creates a beautiful web page for each recipient, and ensures that we all keep boxes of tissue around by sending the most emotional stories to us to keep us focused on why we do what we do. And our assistant, Erin, keeps us on track, running our lives, our calendars, our nonstop travel arrangements, and our dogs.

All of them will tell you they have the "best jobs ever." We think we have the "best staff ever" because we share the same values, we focus on the positive, our gratitude is received with gratitude back to us for all we do to celebrate nurses, and we know we are making a difference. Our team has each other's backs, so when one is out, others pitch in. Without asking how they can help each other, they just help. We do our best to live RADCRAP with Faith, with a special effort on Saturday's Promise—to keep everything in Perspective. (And we are grateful to Joe for referring to Determination rather than Tenacity for Wednesday's Promise.)

We believe in the Invisible Architecture you will now read about and in the tools Bob and Joe propose to create a positive, successful environment for your staff, your patients, and their families. We hope you will find this book an uplifting read and a very effective approach to improving the environment of care in your organization.

Importantly, to all of you who take care of patients or who care for the people who care for patients, we express our gratitude! The work you do is extraordinary. We certainly keep that in perspective every day, and we hope you do, too.

By Bonnie and Mark Barnes, FAANs
Cofounders, The DAISY Foundation™
Honorary members of Sigma Theta Tau International

Part 1

A Culture of Ownership

"

[Growth outliers—organizations that achieve outstanding growth over an extended period of time] focus management attention on culture and shared values. We found (as have others who study high-performing organizations) that the outliers on our list pay close attention to values, culture, and alignment. What does that mean in practice? We saw significant investments in creating an appropriate corporate culture, in employee training, and in executive development among these companies... These organizations invest seriously in corporate values, which their leaders back up through meaningful symbolic actions.

"

—Rita Gunther McGrath:
"How the Growth Outliers Do It"

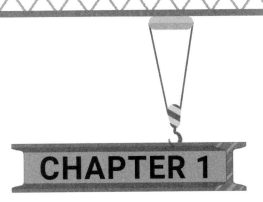

CHAPTER 1

Invisible Architecture

Chapter Goals

- Describe our metaphor for the Invisible Architecture of an organization in which the foundation consists of core values, the superstructure is organizational culture, and the interior finish is workplace attitude.

- Explain why Invisible Architecture is more important than the visible architecture of bricks and mortar in determining the employee experience and the patient experience.

- Describe "the healthcare crisis within" of incivility, bullying, and toxic emotional negativity in the workplace and the way it contributes to stress, burnout, and compassion fatigue.

When a new physical facility is designed, professional architects and engineers guide companies through the process; there are multiple iterations, from schematic design to final construction blueprints; and committees give input on wallpaper design and carpet color. Room designs are laid out with masking tape in the parking lot to ensure a good fit between the new design and the processes and equipment for which that space is being designed. At each step along the way, revisions are made. No detail is left to chance. By the time construction begins, large groups of people will have participated in the design process, creating a clear vision of what the facility will look like.

But when it comes to employee engagement, patient satisfaction, effective communication, and even quality and productivity, the visible architecture of the physical structure is less important than what we call *Invisible Architecture*—the core values, organizational culture, and workplace attitude of an organization. Yet most healthcare organizations do not put nearly as much thought and attention into the design of their Invisible Architecture as they do into the design of their physical facilities. A patient care floor would not be remodeled without a detailed blueprint, but once the remodeling is finished and staff move in, the Invisible Architecture is allowed to evolve haphazardly, with the result that there is cultural fragmentation across the organization. This is one reason that many healthcare organizations have no consistent overarching culture but rather constitute a patchwork of cultures that vary by department, shift, census, staffing level, manager on duty, and other variables. There is a much different culture in nursing than in pharmacy, physical therapy, environmental services, or the business office. And within nursing, there can be quite a different culture on medical-surgical units than in critical care, the emergency department, the surgical suite, or outpatient clinics.

Invisible Architecture is the soul of an organization in the way that bricks and mortar comprise the body of that organization. In recent years, a growing body of empirical research has demonstrated that care of the spirit is just as important to human health and well-being as is care of the body. In the same way, healthcare leaders need to be as deliberate in caring for the soul of the organization as they are in caring for the physical facilities.

When a new building goes up, it is built in three stages: The foundation is put down, a superstructure is erected upon that foundation, and the interior is finished off with carpeting and wallpaper. If you have a good designer and a good builder, the construction is seamless—you don't see where the foundation ends and the superstructure begins, and there are no structural gaps between the walls and the carpeting. We use this construction metaphor to describe Invisible Architecture. The foundation consists of core values, the superstructure is organizational culture, and the interior finish is workplace attitude. As with physical design, in great organizations the transitions are seamless. If, for example, one foundational value of the organization is integrity, it would have a culture that honors confidentiality and personal dignity and a *workplace attitude* that is intolerant of gossip and rumormongering.

From First Impressions to Lasting Impressions

When someone walks into your hospital, your clinic, your long-term care or rehabilitation facility, or your corporate offices, their first impression is created by the physical facilities. A brand-new, well-lit atrium with vaulted ceilings and beautiful artwork on the walls creates a vastly different first impression than a 50-year-old lobby with a low ceiling, fluorescent tube lighting, and aging wallpaper clinging precariously to the drywall.

But that first impression doesn't last long, does it? Someone who has been an inpatient with you for 5 days won't even mention the visible architecture if they're asked about the experience, will they? Rather, they will talk about things that are not physically visible. They'll talk about the way values, explicit and implicit, are reflected, or not reflected, in the actual day-to-day operations of your organization. They'll talk about the culture of the organization, or the corner of the organization they experienced, and how that culture is reflected in relationships. They'll talk about the attitudes and behaviors of the caregivers who treated them. And not just direct caregivers—people from nutrition and environmental services also have a significant impact on the patient experience.

The most successful organizations have attractive and functional physical plants, of course. But they also understand that their greatness derives from things that cannot be seen, not from beautiful buildings or shiny chrome fixtures. They are as diligent in working on their people and culture as they are on their structures and strategies.

The Great Place to Work Institute, which works annually with *Fortune* to create its 100 Best Companies to Work For list, says that the three most important determinants of being a great place to work are pride, connection, and trust. *Note:* These are not qualities that can be developed with business strategy, technology, or physical construction. They are outcomes that spring from the Invisible Architecture of values, culture, and attitude. The best workplaces are more than just places to work—they inspire a spirit of teamwork, a sense of family and fellowship, and a culture of ownership.

Monopoly Cultures

The focus in this book is on healthcare culture in particular, but healthcare organizations can learn and grow by paying attention to what works—and what doesn't work—in other fields. Here are several examples:

- Southwest Airlines flies the same types of airplanes and recruits the same pilots, flight attendants, and mechanics that are employed by every other airline, but has by far the highest employee loyalty and productivity in the industry. With its employment mantra of "Hire for attitude, train for skill," Southwest has redefined the measure of success in the airline industry.

- Zappos sells the same shoes you can buy in any department store, but getting a job at its call center is more competitive than trying to get into Harvard University. The company went from start-up to a billion-dollar enterprise in 8 years, and has created a tremendous competitive advantage from promoting its culture and the 10 core values on which that culture is built.

- Les Schwab sells the same tires you can buy at any other tire store; Schwab came to dominate the tire business in the Pacific Northwest by creating an empire of people "on fire to sell you a tire." (An employee actually runs out to your car to welcome you when you pull into the parking lot.)

- Starbucks built a global powerhouse in less than two decades selling the ultimate commodity product—coffee—at a substantial premium over what people could get it for from a Folgers can. When the company got into serious trouble in 2008, it was its resilient culture, more than any brilliant strategies, that set the stage for one of the most impressive business turnarounds ever.

Examples taken from *The Cultural Blueprinting Toolkit Workbook* by Joe Tye; used with permission.

Every organization that makes "Best Companies" and "Great Places to Work" rosters intuitively understands that the Invisible Architecture of core values, organizational culture, and emotional attitude creates the only self-sustaining source of competitive advantage. You might not have a monopoly on your market, but you do have a monopoly on your *culture*. Strategy can be copied, technology can be leapfrogged, and your best people can be recruited away by competitors. But no one can steal your values, copy your culture, or compete with your attitude. Every culture is unique, but some cultures are, as the saying goes, more unique than others. Designing and building a beautiful, singular Invisible Architecture is one of the most immediately rewarding things a leader can do, and one of the greatest legacies that person can leave.

The Foundation of Core Values

A culture of ownership rests on the foundation of the organization's core values. Ken Blanchard (1999, p. 175), coauthor of *The One-Minute Manager* and a leading authority on organizational excellence, couldn't be more accurate when he says, "Identifying the core values that define your organization is one of the most important functions of leadership. The success or failure of this process can literally make or break an organization." Think of core values as the acorn of an organization. It's easy to admire the majesty and grandeur of an oak tree without giving a single thought to such a tiny, seemingly insignificant thing as the seed it once was—but you'll never see an oak tree that didn't start out as an acorn. Every great organization has a great set of core values embedded within its DNA.

Whether it's for an individual or an organization, a statement of core values should help to define who you are, what you stand for, and what you won't stand for. (And, as the old country song says, if you don't stand for something, you'll fall for anything.) At the personal level, a *core value* is a deeply held philosophical commitment that defines and shapes how you think, how you set goals and make decisions, how you develop relationships, and how you deal with conflict. At the organizational level, a core value should define non-negotiable expectations regarding how people behave, the goals toward which they direct their collective efforts, and how they work together. People will act on an organization's values only to the extent that they perceive them to be congruent with their personal values. In Chapter 8, we go into greater detail about the interconnection of personal and organizational values.

The Superstructure of Organizational Culture

Any time you walk through a building's front doors, you are surrounded by superstructure. The building swallows you up.

The same concept holds true for the superstructure of the Invisible Architecture: culture. Every organization has a culture, though in many cases that culture has evolved without careful, or even conscious, design.

Culture is to the organization what personality is to the individual. A culture, like a person, can be warm and caring, callous and domineering, or shallow and money-hungry, for example. And, like a personality, a culture always reflects a set of core values, either consciously or unconsciously. Your core cultural characteristics will inevitably shape the image of your organization, your *brand*, in the public's perception.

It's a common misconception that culture is not amenable to leadership influence. There are, in fact, many examples of massive and rapid changes being made, for better or worse.

The Veterans Health Administration offers examples of both good and bad cultural changes. During the 1970s and '80s, VHA hospitals were widely perceived as places for eligible residents to go for care if they could not afford "real," nonmilitary hospitals, and where clinicians who weren't sufficiently competent to be admitted to the medical staffs of those real hospitals went to practice. Then, during the mid-1990s, Dr. Kenneth W. Kizer oversaw a profound cultural transformation that, within the span of several years, changed a culture that had accepted mediocrity into a culture that demands excellence (Longman, 2012). Dr. Kizer engaged the directors of all 172 (at that time) VHA medical centers in a dialogue about core values; after extensive interaction, these were defined as trust, respect, excellence, commitment, and compassion.

More recently, a military-style command-and-control regime issued a new statement of core values—integrity, commitment, accountability, respect, and excellence (ICARE)—with minimal input from the field. At the time, many caregivers balked at being told that compassion was suddenly no longer a core value of the Veterans Health Administration. This top-down approach to management contributed to a culture of blame-shifting and in some cases outright cheating. Rather than own up to problems that contributed to severe scheduling delays and make a good-faith effort to fix these problems, as would happen in a healthy and productive culture, some managers fudged the numbers, resulting in a scandal that has tarnished the reputation of the entire system.

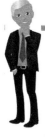

A Note from Joe

Values Coach has worked with more than a dozen Veterans Health Administration facilities, and I am consistently impressed with the spirit of ownership reflected by the professionals who work in these organizations, most of whom refer to the people they serve as "our veterans" or "my veterans," and not just as "the veterans." It is sad to see so many wonderful people tarnished by a scandal rooted in a flawed culture. ■

Every organization is truly a cultural patchwork quilt. Ideally, a few overarching themes define the overarching culture of the organization, which are then woven into the subculture of each different unit. When cultural norms are clear, there is less need for rule-based accountability to enforce behavioral expectations.

The Interior Finish of Emotional Attitude

Most building interiors are tastefully finished: taupe walls, gray carpet, maybe some blue trim, a wood accent here and there. They are pleasant but dull. Try to remember what the ceiling of your childhood home looked like. Was it white? Off-white? Somewhere in between?

Now think of the ceiling of the Sistine Chapel, or Grand Central Station. It doesn't happen often, but the finish of a building can take your breath away.

Attitudes are like that. Some are mundane and forgettable, whereas others are empowering and inspiring.

In recent years, much has been written about *emotional intelligence*, a term popularized by Daniel Goleman (1995); being emotionally intelligent means recognizing your emotions for what they are, interpreting them correctly, and weeding out self-defeating dispositions and behaviors. If we had to encapsulate the whole complex phenomenon of emotional intelligence in a single word, it would be this: *positivity*.

Emotional positivity is essential to a culture of ownership. People with an ownership mindset are cheerful and optimistic at work. A culture of ownership cannot exist in an environment where people are disgusted with their jobs, resentful of their bosses, and hostile to their colleagues. Some workplaces permanently seem to convey the feeling that a tragic event has just happened and a catastrophe is right around the corner. One key duty of a leadership team—and one that is too often ignored or abdicated—is to confront toxic emotional negativity and establish an expectation that employees will have positive attitudes at work and will treat others with respect. Leaders owe this to their customers and to their more positive employees. For that matter, they owe it to their negative employees as well because negativity is, in most cases, a clear symptom of deep-rooted unhappiness.

Toxic emotional negativity isn't anything mysterious or exotic. You've probably experienced it one way or another. Have you ever been ignored or treated dismissively by an indifferent bureaucrat? Walked into a break room where the resident emotional vampire is holding court? Have you ever tried to have a meaningful conversation with a truculent teenager who is in a bad mood? If your answer to any of these questions is yes, you know what toxic emotional negativity is.

Toxic emotional negativity is our name for the whole collection of behaviors—gossiping, eye-rolling, bullying, and work-shirking, for example—that people use to register their contempt for their organizations, their coworkers, and the people they are there to serve (and are being paid to serve). Coworkers who secretly (or not so secretly) think that their jobs, their peers, their customers, and even their bosses are beneath them—that in doing their work they are suffering some unspeakable indignity (usually, they presume, with the patience of a saint)—are reflecting toxic emotional negativity. They engage in behaviors that are, in ways subtle and not so subtle, harmful to others. In fact, such behaviors have recently been labeled as *microaggressions*.

Toxic emotional negativity is so ubiquitous that you hardly even notice it unless you're making a concerted effort to do so—but that doesn't mean it can't harm you. To the contrary, it is the emotional and spiritual equivalent of cigarette smoke in the air. Secondhand negativity can be as harmful to the spirit as secondhand smoke is to the body. One or two emotional vampires can poison an entire workplace, dragging down the morale and the productivity of everyone around them. You cannot help but be influenced by the people you spend time with. Being chronically subjected to toxic emotional negativity in the workplace contributes to stress, burnout, compassion fatigue, and other harmful emotional states. And the baleful impact is not limited to the workplace; you are likely to take these secondhand emotions home and infect your families with them.

You've undoubtedly heard the expression "Misery loves company." It simply means this: Miserable people go out of their way to make everyone they come in contact with miserable, too. That's why it is called *commiserating*: To commiserate means to be miserable together! So, toxic emotional negativity spreads like an infection. In the 19th century, doctors didn't wash their hands before they performed surgery; no one knew what a germ was, so no one saw the need. Imagine if an emotional revolution in healthcare could happen as sweeping and profound as sanitization brought to physical care. In fact, the soul and the body are not so disconnected—conclusive evidence now shows that negative emotions are physically harmful. It is a core leadership responsibility to create a workplace environment where toxic emotional negativity is not tolerated. This is especially true in healthcare, where toxic emotional negativity in the workplace can also cause iatrogenic (hospital-induced) anxiety for patients.

The emotional climate of the workplace is defined by behaviors you expect and behaviors you tolerate; over time, the behaviors you tolerate will dominate the behaviors you say you expect. If leaders *say they expect* cheerful customer service but then *tolerate* toxic emotional negativity, it becomes the accepted standard. If leaders *say they expect* respect but then *tolerate* people gossiping about others behind their backs, respect for the dignity of others becomes only a good intention. When leaders tolerate behaviors that violate the organization's professed core values, the predictable result is that the expectation of integrity is perched on a slippery slope that ends with "never get caught" instead of "always do the right thing" as the accepted standard.

This Building Is Never Finished

When construction on a new healthcare facility is finished, there's usually a celebratory ceremony. Somebody with clout—the CEO or maybe a governor—says a few words before cutting a symbolic ribbon with a giant pair of scissors. The crowd applauds politely. Sometimes there's wine and cheese. The building is finished!

But is it, really? What if, from the moment the ribbon is cut, everyone acts like the building *is* finished? What if no one ever mows the grass, or polishes the windows, or mops the floors? What if the supply closets are never restocked? What if the equipment is never recalibrated, let alone upgraded? If you walked in to work tomorrow and found that your hospital had downsized every janitor, landscaper, clerk, and technician on the payroll, how long could it keep providing patients with quality care? If you leave a building alone long enough, it starts to fall apart.

In the same way, work on Invisible Architecture never ends. One essential responsibility of leadership is to maintain cultural momentum. New employees must be oriented to the values, culture, and attitudinal expectations of the organization. Policies and procedures that are no longer helpful must be phased out and new ones established (as many organizations recently found out with regard to cellphones and social media). Managers at all levels must be vigilant that their own attitudes and behaviors are setting the right example and that people in their organization, or their areas of the organization, are following that example. Changes in technology, the competitive playing field, and societal expectations will all influence the Invisible Architecture of the organization. There is always more work to be done—but as long as you're doing the right kind of work, you will find reasons for celebration. A healthy culture is self-sustaining and, in many ways, even self-directing.

The Healthcare Crisis Within

Incivility. Disrespect. Bullying. Lateral or horizontal violence. "Nurses eat their young." The prevalence of terms and phrases like these in the healthcare literature in general and the nursing literature in particular suggests that "the healthcare crisis" consists of not only what is happening in the external environment but also reflects a healthcare crisis within. Ever since Florence Nightingale's revolutionary contributions to the field, healthcare has been defined by its singular ability to balance scientific precision with a spirit of compassionate care. As the pace of change continues to accelerate, it is ever more important that you care for that spirit: "Nightingale's enduring legacy is socially relevant because the profession of nursing shows signs of losing its soul; it is in crisis" (Dossey, 2005, p. xiii). It is time to revive the soul that has always made the profession of healing great.

An organization that has a reputation for a negative emotional environment will find it increasingly difficult to recruit and retain good people, especially in the nursing profession. Over the next 10 years, an estimated one-third of practicing nurses will retire. To replace these individuals, more than a million new nurses will need to enter the profession. The competition will be intense. Organizations that have a reputation for having a positive culture of ownership will attract and retain the best talent, and others will be forced to resort to temporary staffing agencies and paying extraordinary hiring bonuses in their efforts to recruit new staff and replace those who leave.

Summary

The first impression patients and visitors have of your organization will be created by the visible architecture of brick and mortar, carpeting, and wallpaper. But the lasting impression will be determined by things that are felt more than seen— the Invisible Architecture. Values Coach uses a construction metaphor for Invisible Architecture in which the foundation is core values, the superstructure is organizational culture, and the interior finish is workplace attitude. Just as the physical facility must be continuously maintained and periodically upgraded, so too the Invisible Architecture requires routine maintenance and occasional overhaul.

Chapter Questions

- Does your organization have a cultural blueprint (or equivalent) for its Invisible Architecture?

- Who in your organization should be engaged in the cultural blueprinting process?

- Does your organization's Invisible Architecture of core values, organizational culture, and workplace attitude serve to differentiate you from your competitors for recruiting and retention, patient loyalty, and community reputation?

- If employees in your organization saw a billboard promoting it as a great place to work, would they nod their heads in proud agreement or would they roll their eyes in disbelief?

References

Blanchard, K. H. (1999). *The heart of a leader.* Tulsa, OK: Honor Books.

Dossey, B. M. (2005). *Florence Nightingale today: Healing, leadership, global action.* Silver Spring, MD: American Nurses Association.

Goleman, D. (1995). *Emotional intelligence.* New York, NY: Bantam Books.

Longman, P. (2012). *Best care anywhere: Why VA health care would work better for everyone.* Oakland, CA: Berrett-Koehler Publishers.

> **"**
>
> *Accountability is supposed to improve productivity by tracking performance. Up to a point, like most well-intentioned management expectations, this one may have the desired effect. In the long run, however, there could hardly be a more inhibiting practice. When made a fetish, accountability stifles creativity. Far from making employees perform better long term, accountability encourages a culture of evasion, denial, and finger pointing.*
>
> **"**
>
> —Richard Farson and Ralph Keyes,
> *The Innovation Paradox*

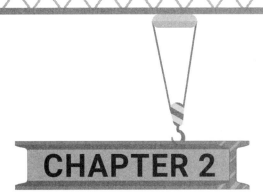

From Accountability to Ownership

Chapter Goals

- Describe the three levels of the accountability continuum, what you can and cannot hold people accountable for, and the downside of fostering a culture of hierarchical accountability.

- Describe six reasons why a culture that relies on hierarchical accountability for performance management will inevitably underperform.

- Explain why "the right bus" is the wrong metaphor, and why a much more appropriate metaphor is "the galley ship."

- Explain why healthcare organizations should transition from a culture of accountability to a culture of ownership.

No one ever changes the oil in a rental car. Most people return the car with a full gas tank because doing so is specified in the contract—they are accountable for it. But no one washes and waxes the car or checks the transmission fluid, because no one feels pride of ownership in a car that belongs to a faceless corporation. When you move from a culture of mere accountability to a culture of ownership, you create a sustainable source of competitive advantage for both recruiting and retaining great people and for earning long-term patient loyalty.

Accountability is doing what *you are supposed to do* because someone else expects it of you; it springs from the extrinsic motivation of reward and punishment. The *Merriam-Webster Dictionary* definition of accountability is:

> *Subject to having to report, explain or justify; being answerable, responsible.*

An organization that seeks to promote accountability according to this definition will likely end up with a workplace where people do only the tasks that are listed in their job descriptions and never take initiative or go above and beyond the tasks they are being held accountable for. Perhaps worse, there is likely to be a diminished sense of pride in the work itself when it is being done for the expectation of reward or the fear of punishment.

Accountability is extrinsic motivation—being answerable to someone else. Not only can you not hold people accountable for the tasks that really matter, but an excessive focus on accountability also has a real downside. Trying to hold people accountable achieves only a short-term rise in results that quickly deteriorates into another "program of the month" that comes and goes without creating a sustained impact on the cultural DNA of the organization.

Ownership is doing *what needs to be done* because you expect it of yourself; ownership springs from the intrinsic motivation of pride and engagement. The dictionary definition of ownership is:

> *The state, relation, or fact of being an owner, which in turn is defined as to have power or mastery over.*

A culture in which all employees are encouraged to think like an owner and to have mastery over their work will inevitably outperform an accountability-driven organization in every dimension that truly matters, including employee engagement, productivity, customer service, recruiting and retention success, and profitability.

Leaders need to hold employees accountable for fulfilling the terms of their job descriptions, and for behaving in ways that are consistent with the values and mission of that organization. But in today's turbulent and hypercompetitive world, that's not enough to remain competitive, much less to make the now proverbial jump "from good to great." Employees in great organizations hold themselves and each other to higher standards of expectation for their attitudes and behaviors as well as for their performance at work. They have pride of ownership.

In the course of working with healthcare clients, Joe often hears people say, "We don't hold each other accountable." But when he presses the issue, they're usually not talking about accountability—they're talking about ownership; they are really saying that people don't take ownership for their work, their results, and their relationships—and because they are not holding themselves accountable, someone else must do it. So it's important to distinguish those factors for which employees can be held accountable through managerial discipline or intimidation and those factors for which they cannot be held accountable but which must be accomplished through personal ownership.

You can hold employees accountable for this:	But not for this:
Complying with rules	Living values
Showing up on time	Being emotionally present
Discipline	Loyalty
Saying the right words	Asking the right questions
Meeting budgets	Thinking entrepreneurially
Meeting deadlines	Working with passion
Results	Dreams
Competence	Caring
What they say at work	What they say at home
Appearance	Pride
Treating people with respect	Honoring people's dignity
Saluting	Laughing
Their job descriptions	Their life decisions

The Three Levels of Accountability

Numbers can tell you a lot, but they can't tell you everything. Counting calories isn't an effective way to manage your health if your diet is high in arsenic. W. Edwards Deming, the guru of Total Quality Management, said that what gets measured gets done, and he encouraged clients to find ways to quantify every important parameter of the operation. But Deming also said that the most important characteristics of your organization cannot be counted. How does one inventory pride or measure enthusiasm? You can certainly *see* these qualities in people's attitudes and behaviors in the best of organizations, but they are steadfastly resistant to quantification.

There are three levels of accountability: hierarchical, cultural, and personal. This concept is especially important for leaders in hospitals and other healthcare organizations to understand because you cannot hold people hierarchically accountable for the things that truly matter in the healing professions. You cannot promote caring and compassion, pride and loyalty, or enthusiasm and fellowship by strictly enforcing a code of conduct or by using disciplinary action to hold employees accountable. In that respect, mere accountability establishes a very low bar for performance expectations. The accountability continuum can be seen as a 3-tiered pyramid, as shown in Figure 2.1.

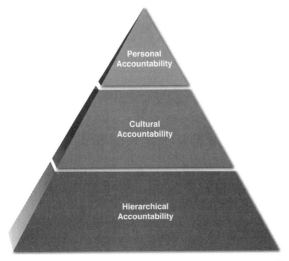

Figure 2.1   *This 3-tiered pyramid shows the different levels of accountability.*

Hierarchical accountability (management)

At the lowest level, *hierarchical* accountability is top-down command-and-control. It's what people typically mean when they use the word *accountability*. It is reward and punishment, looking over people's shoulders, and holding their feet to the fire (a term that originated from a medieval form of torture).

Hierarchical accountability works especially well in tightly regimented, bureaucratic organizations. The factory worker who misses a quota is docked by the floor manager; the mail clerk who forgets to file a form is sanctioned by the supervisor; a high school math teacher holds students accountable for doing their homework every night by threatening to flunk them at the end of the semester; the teacher in turn is held accountable for students achieving certain scores on standardized tests.

In healthcare contexts, hierarchical accountability is most appropriate for tasks that have significant potential for harm. Employees must be held accountable for administering the proper medications to patients, for completing safety checklists before surgery, and if they are managers for hitting productivity and budgetary targets. They must be held accountable for behaviors that cause harm: theft, bullying, and malicious gossip must have consequences.

Managers often find, to their dismay, that trying to hold people accountable might achieve short-term gains in whatever element is being counted (the word *accountable* means "able to be counted") but, in fairly short order, backsliding begins. A customer service initiative may get off to a good start, with employees being given a script and a happy-face pin and then being held accountable for saying the words. But it soon becomes obvious to patients that some people are simply parroting the script and not speaking from the heart. What the manager is measuring (whether every predetermined word is rattled off in the correct order) is quite different from what patients perceive (a soulless, boring rendition of rules and regulations undertaken from a resentful sense of obligation).

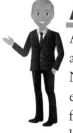

A Note from Bob

As a patient in my own organization, I got out of bed to ambulate soon after surgery. I was in mild pain and had an NG tube still in place. My wife was at my side. If you've ever had an NG tube in place, you know it is not comfortable and, of course, doesn't look good either. In the hallway, I was approached by two nurse managers I know well; I would even consider them friends. I cracked a smile and began having a conversation with them. Then, one manager pulled out her iPad and said she needed to ask some questions about my stay. She began her list of questions. The conversation turned from personal to impersonal quickly. But this was the process we had established to capture data and to assure that our leaders were rounding consistently. If I didn't like it, what did other patients think?

Soon after this experience, we stopped the scripting and asked each leader to be authentic; to be personable. In a culture of ownership, leaders accept responsibility for patients' and visitors' experience. Many stories have been shared in which leaders do extraordinary things to make sure patients are having an exceptional care experience. ■

Cultural accountability (peers)

Cultural accountability is peer pressure, in the broadest sense of that term. It is far more powerful than hierarchical accountability, for better and worse. In many organizations, cultural accountability exerts a negative pressure on productivity and performance, such as when someone experiences peer pressure against being an overachiever, a quota-buster, or a brown-noser. Attempting to impose hierarchical accountability for customer service excellence in a toxically negative culture requires far more energy than achieving the same outcome with cultural accountability, and is much more likely to fail, because of the inevitable passive-aggressive resistance. Trying to change culture is much harder than merely trying to impose rules, though it is much more likely to achieve a sustained impact.

Perhaps the best example of the power of cultural accountability is the way that enforcement of nonsmoking policies has changed over the years. Hospitals no longer require no-smoking signs in every room, and managers almost never have to discipline employees for sneaking a smoke on the job. Why? Because cultural expectations have changed so profoundly over the past several decades. Anyone lighting a cigarette on an airplane today would not need to be arrested by an air marshal as much as they would need to be rescued from fellow passengers. (Healthcare organizations have much to learn from the movement to abolish smoking in public places, as we explain in Chapter 10.)

Personal accountability (self)

Personal accountability is the highest and best form of accountability. People who accept personal accountability don't need someone else looking over their shoulders or coworkers pressuring them into behaving in a certain manner—they do it because it's a reflection of their personal values.

Building a culture of ownership often entails a gradual transition from hierarchical to cultural, and then to personal accountability. Personal accountability, the foundation of a culture of ownership, comes from within, not from above.

At most airlines, flight attendants believe that they've completed the job once they've parroted the script about seat belts and oxygen masks, whether or not people are actually listening (which, in most cases, they are not). The attendants have passed the test of hierarchical accountability. At Southwest Airlines, on the other hand, flight attendants recognize that the *real* job isn't simply parroting the script—it's making sure that passengers hear it. When David Holmes presents the words of the script as a rap song or Marty Cobb presents it as a comedy routine, people not only listen, they also give the flight attendant a round of applause. When someone records the performance with a cellphone and the video goes viral, Southwest benefits from millions of dollars' worth of free advertising.

A culture of ownership provides an unbeatable source of competitive advantage. United Airlines has a culture of accountability; Southwest Airlines has a culture of ownership. Walmart has a culture of accountability; Costco has a culture of ownership. Hertz has a culture of accountability; Enterprise has a culture of ownership. Payless Shoes has a culture of accountability; Zappos has a culture of ownership. In each of these cases, the company with a culture of ownership is winning the competitive battle.

Why Accountability Isn't Enough

Make no mistake: All three levels of accountability are indispensable in any organization. Accountants must be accountable for getting the math right; nurses must be accountable for giving the proper medications to patients; housekeepers must be accountable for keeping the place clean. The real question is whether they *hold themselves* accountable (a culture of ownership) or need to be held accountable by a boss (a culture of accountability). A culture of ownership is not created by economic interest; it springs from emotional commitment. When people feel a sense of ownership for the work, they don't need to be held accountable for doing their jobs.

Many organizations have put quite a bit of effort into various initiatives to hold people accountable, often with dismaying results. After an initial improvement in whatever measure they're trying to hold people accountable for achieving (patient or customer satisfaction, productivity, or sales, for example), things go back to the way they were before the program. Sometimes, they even get worse.

The following sections spell out seven reasons why a focus on accountability can end up being counterproductive.

Reason #1: Accountability implies irresponsibility

When you tell people that you're going to hold them accountable for something, it sends a subtle but unmistakable message that you don't believe they can be trusted to hold *themselves* accountable. The IRS holds people accountable for filing their taxes by April 15 because it knows that they can't be trusted to do it voluntarily. But no one needs to be held accountable for making it to the dock on time to board a cruise ship. Homeowners mow their lawns because they have pride of ownership; renters need to be held accountable for hiring someone else to cut the grass. People who take pride in their work, their organizations, their professions, and themselves don't need to be held accountable for memorizing a script to provide great customer service or compassionate patient care. They do it because they are intrinsically motivated, not because someone is forcing them or coercing them.

Reason #2: Holding people accountable can be exhausting

It takes a lot of management energy to hold people accountable. The more time and energy a manager must spend holding people accountable, the less time and energy that manager has for the more creative and productive work of leadership. You can think of it as "accountability fatigue."

Reason #3: Accountability focuses on rules, not on values

People cannot be held accountable for commitment, enthusiasm, passion, pride, or caring. These qualities must come from an inner conviction, an intrinsic sense of ownership. You don't hold people accountable for living values; you hold them accountable for following rules. When people share in a common set of values, you don't need to set a lot of rules. The Nordstrom department store chain is famous for customer service excellence. In HR circles, the company is also famous for its two-sentence policy manual, which simply says: "At Nordstrom we only have one rule. Use good judgment in all situations." Nordstrom employees don't need to be held accountable for going above and beyond the terms of their job descriptions. They do it because they have taken ownership of the work.

Reason #4: Accountability is always after the fact and often demotivating

You empower people to do the things that need to be done in the future; you hold people accountable for the things that have, or have not, been done in the past. You can empower a nurse to practice at the top of her professional capabilities, and you hold her accountable when she fails the test. You can motivate a salesperson to make calls; you hold him accountable for not making those calls. Imagine going home at the end of the day and saying to your family: "Today I was held accountable for. . . ." Can you think of anything—anything at all—that would allow you to finish that sentence in a way that would make your family proud of you and motivate you to go to work tomorrow with a little more swagger in your step?

An excessive focus on accountability can be particularly harmful when it comes to performance appraisals—especially if the appraisals are performed only quarterly or, worse, annually, or if the evaluating manager has a span of control that is too large to allow a truly valid assessment. "Annual reviews," note Cappelli and Tavis (2016), "hold people accountable for past behaviors at the expense of improving current performance and grooming talent for the future, both of which are critical for organizations' long-term survival."

Reason #5: You cannot hold people accountable for loyalty

Ownership is, we've come to believe, the "secret sauce" that the most successful organizations have. It both creates a sustainable competitive advantage for recruiting and retaining great people and for earning the lifelong loyalty of customers. These organizations earn what loyalty expert Fred Reichheld (2003) calls *barnacles*, or, in other words, "customers who are likely to stick around for a lifetime" (p. 88). You cannot hold either employees or customers accountable for being loyal to the organization—that only comes from a spirit of ownership.

Reason #6: Excessive focus on accountability can provide an incentive to cheat

More than 40 years ago, sociologist Donald Campbell and economist Charles Goodhart concluded from research in their own professions that when a performance measure is turned into a performance target, it ceases to be a good measure, largely because it can inadvertently incentivize perverse behavior. This syndrome shows up repeatedly in the organizational world: Managers at Sears auto repair shops selling people muffler systems that they didn't need; Wells Fargo agents establishing bank accounts and credit cards for people who didn't request them; and Veterans Health Administration managers falsifying appointment wait-time records—the examples are endless.

Reason #7: Accountability will never take an organization from good to great

If you read *Fortune* magazine's annual listings of America's most admired companies and America's 100 best companies to work for, you will see that not one of these organizations earned a place on these rosters by promoting a culture of accountability. To be sure, they all have standards of behavior and performance to which people are held accountable, but they all appreciate that these are minimal standards—they are the price of entry for being in business. Going from good to great requires a culture of ownership.

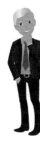

A Note from Joe

When I was an inpatient for one week at the University of Iowa Hospitals and Clinics with acute diverticulitis, four registered nurses were primarily responsible for my care. By the time I was discharged, I had completed four nominations for DAISY Awards, one for each of those nurses. (Participating hospitals encourage patients to nominate nurses who go above and beyond the call of duty—see more at www.daisyfoundation.org.) Not one of those nominations was completed because the nurse was doing an excellent job at something she could be held accountable for, something included in the RN job description. In each case, it was for going above and beyond the basic elements of the job description—of doing the sorts of things that people who own the work will do that people who are "renting a spot" on the organization chart will not do. ∎

Summary

In its most common usage, the word "accountability" refers to the top-down accountability of reward and punishment. A culture that depends upon hierarchical accountability is subject to unintended consequences that can harm service quality and productivity. Cultural accountability is the peer-to-peer process of employees holding each other accountable for certain standards of behavior. For better or worse, it is often more influential than hierarchical accountability. The highest level is personal accountability, where employees hold themselves accountable and do not need bosses or coworkers looking over their shoulders. Personal accountability is the basis for a culture of ownership, which is one of the most powerful sources of competitive advantage an organization can gain.

Chapter Questions

- Which of the three levels of the accountability continuum is most prevalent in your organization?
- Which of the three levels of the accountability continuum do you respond to? Which do you personally find to be most motivating—hierarchical, cultural, or personal?
- Within your organization (or your family), which activities are most appropriately managed by hierarchical, cultural, and personal accountability?
- How far along on the journey from accountability to ownership is your organization, and what can be done to move it further along?

References

Cappelli, P., & Tavis, A. (2016, Oct.). The performance management revolution. *Harvard Business Review*. Retrieved from https://hbr.org/2016/10/the-performance-management-revolution

Farson, R. E., & Keyes, R. (2003). *The innovation paradox: The success of failure, the failure of success.* New York, NY: Free Press.

Reichheld, F. (2003). *Loyalty rules: How today's leaders build lasting relationships.* Boston, MA: Harvard Business School Press.

Part 2

The Invisible Architecture

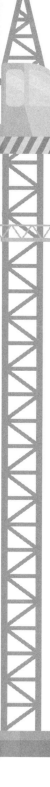

"

Every excellent company we studied is clear on what it stands for, and takes the process of value shaping seriously. In fact, we wonder whether it is possible to be an excellent company without clarity on values and without having the right sorts of values.

"

–Tom Peters and Bob Waterman,
In Search of Excellence

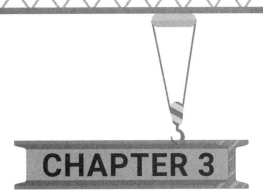

The Foundation of Core Values

Chapter Goals

- Describe the ideal statement of values and explain why the values statements of many healthcare organizations do not effectively inspire employees or create competitive distinction in the marketplace.

- Describe the Values > Behaviors > Outcomes continuum and explain why it is important for motivating the behaviors that are required to achieve valued outcomes.

- Discuss the importance of coherence between the posted values of the organization and the internalized personal values of the individual.

- Discuss the importance of core values in times of adversity and the acid test of living your values.

A *statement of values* is, or should be, the single most important document in your organization; it is, or should be, the set of guiding principles that defines cultural norms and performance expectations. Even your organization's vision and mission statements should be rooted in the underpinning core values. This is because any mission you can devise and any vision you can foresee will ultimately be a reflection, or a projection, of core values. In the Invisible Architecture model of an organization, those values are the foundation on which the superstructure of organizational culture rests and the interior finish of workplace attitude is built.

An effective statement of values defines who you are, what you stand for, and what you won't stand for.

A powerful statement of values that is embraced by everyone in the organization is an essential element of a culture of ownership. The organization's core values should be introduced in the recruiting process, reinforced in new employee orientation, and revitalized in staff meetings, in nursing unit huddles, and at other opportunities on an ongoing basis. And there should be an expectation that employees know these values by heart (not just by rote memorization—*by heart*). This is especially true for members of the management team. To be blunt about it, not expecting employees to know the core values of an organization by heart sells them short with the assumption that they either are not smart enough or do not care enough to make the effort. Five-year olds can memorize complex songs like "The Fifty Nifty United States," so healthcare executives should expect employees to know the core values of the organization and to be able to talk intelligently about what those values mean at a personal level. Unfortunately, in many organizations, only a relatively small number of employees actually know the core values by heart (and they aren't always the ones with the word "chief" in their job titles).

A climate of permissive indifference to whether employees really *know* the core values can profoundly undermine the performance potential of the organization. An employee engagement survey completed by Modern Survey (2013) found a direct and powerful correlation between employees having internalized the organization's values and their being engaged in the workplace. According to Modern Survey president Don MacPherson, "Employees who can say they know and understand their organizational values are 30 times more likely to be fully engaged than those who can't say the same. A simple thing like well-communicated organizational values is foundational to creating a culture of engagement" (p. 4). It is, MacPherson says, "shocking" that, given the evidence, leaders don't do more to create an expectation that their employees will know and embrace the organization's core values.

In their work on applying the lessons of military strategy in business leadership, Sullivan and Harper (1996) emphasized the operational significance of values shared by troops of all ranks and levels: "One of the most important lessons we learned during the rebuilding of the Army after Vietnam was the importance of values—a commitment by all soldiers to something larger than themselves" (p. 57).

Culture is the link between values and behaviors (which we'll talk more about in Chapters 4–7). Taking values seriously means that employees are held to the high standards implicit in living those values. For example, it is not possible for someone to be a negative, bitter, cynical, sarcastic emotional vampire in the break room and then somehow flip an inner switch and become genuinely caring and compassionate when dealing with a patient; if that does happen, patients see right through the fraud. If, for example, one of your core values is integrity (and we certainly hope it is, either explicitly or implicitly) but your culture tolerates a rumor mill where employees talk about coworkers behind their backs without being reprimanded, you have set a low bar in your definition of what integrity really means.

The Ideal Statement of Values

A statement of values should, ideally, serve three purposes: Establish the organizational identity, define key functional parameters, and create a focus on operational and societal relevance. We discuss each of these purposes in the following sections.

Organizational identity

A statement of values should help you define, either implicitly or explicitly, the following three characteristics:

- **Who you are:** A great statement of values is the underpinning of brand identity. Everything Disney does is intended to reinforce its self-defined identity as "The Happiest Place On Earth."

Volvo identifies itself as the maker of the world's safest cars. Procter & Gamble (P&G) has five core values that are reinforced by 17 supporting statements; these are further amplified by eight operating principles that have 23 supporting statements. (In case you're counting, that's a total of 53 statements that P&G's leadership believes are needed to fully define who they are, what they stand for, and what they won't stand for.) The preamble to the P&G statement of values simply says: "P&G is its people and the values by which we live." The company includes "Winning" as a core value to undergird its identity as a tough competitor. The P&G statement of values

> " The importance of values in creating clarity and enabling a company to become healthy cannot be overstated. More than anything else, values are critical because they define a company's personality. They provide employees with clarity about how to behave, which reduces the need for inefficient and demoralizing micromanagement.
>
> –Patrick Lencioni: *The Advantage: Why Organizational Health Trumps Everything Else in Business* "

is not boilerplate and has not been dumbed down to fit on the back of a business card; these values and principles are not just warm-and-fuzzy good intentions—they establish a high bar of performance expectations.

- **What you stand for:** The guiding principle of Mary Kay Ash in starting her company was to provide women with the opportunity to set their priorities as God first, family second, and career third. The guiding principle behind Habitat for Humanity is that no one anywhere on earth should have to live in a shack. Catholic Health Initiatives includes "Reverence" as a core value to define expectations about the spirit with which employees treat patients and each other.

  One of the core values of Griffin Hospital in Derby, Connecticut, is entrepreneurship and innovation, which is defined as, "Encouraging and recognizing performance leading to the development of 'value added' programs and services and improvements in efficiency and effectiveness" (Mission & values, n.d.). Through its sponsorship of Planetree, the hospital has had an impact on promoting patient-centered care around the world that is far out of proportion to the size of the hospital itself.

- **What you won't stand for:** The first two of the ten core values of Auto-Owners Insurance Company are honesty and loyalty. The company will not stand for dishonesty and insists on bilateral loyalty. In its 100-year history, it has never had a layoff and is committed to creating opportunities for its associates, but also expects associates to be loyal to the company. It defines *loyalty* as passion, pride, and commitment—not mere tenure. And it is made clear to all associates that if they are ever placed in a position where they are forced to choose between honesty and loyalty—the position in which thousands of Enron employees once found themselves—they are to choose honesty, whatever the cost. Chairman and CEO Jeff Harrold meets with new employees 6 months after their start dates; one of the questions he asks is, "How have you seen our ten core values being acted out in the daily operations of our company?"

Functional parameters

An ideal statement of values should also address these functional parameters:

- Create performance expectations: SSM Health, one of the nation's largest healthcare systems, was the first healthcare organization to earn the Malcolm Baldrige National Quality Award. One of its five core values is "Excellence," which states: "We expect the best of ourselves and one another." SSM's now-retired CEO Sister Mary Jean Ryan describes how raising the bar on performance expectations was crucial to winning that award (2007, p. 104): "Leaders assume responsibility for what happens in their area of work. They 'own' their work and perform a job with integrity, as an expression of themselves, their creativity, and their commitment."

- Establish an emotional connection: Procter & Gamble's core value "Passion for Winning" is clearly intended to attract and motivate people with a strong competitive spirit. Clickstop's (Clickstop Core Values, n.d.) core value of "Make time for fun and family" conveys the message that work and fun aren't mutually exclusive while also honoring the importance of a rewarding life outside of work.

- Catalyze action: The first of the ten core values at Zappos (About Zappos culture, n.d.) is "Deliver WOW through service," which is reinforced by such policies as no time limit or quota being imposed on the company's call center employees. According to Zappos CEO Tony Hsieh, the record length for a call with a single customer was close to 8 hours. In most call center operations, that employee would have been disciplined or terminated. At Zappos that person was celebrated for customer service excellence.

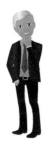

A Note from Joe

I once had a speaking schedule that kept me on the road for a full month without once returning home to repack a suitcase. Midway through the trip, I needed a new pair of running shoes. I ordered them from the Zappos website. When they arrived at my hotel, they were the wrong size, so I called the Zappos call center and spoke with Mary Ann. (When was the last time you remembered the name of a call center employee?) She arranged to have another pair shipped for arrival the next day at the hotel where I would be staying. Then, noticing that I was from Iowa, she said that "we Hawkeyes need to stick together" and that she was going to make me a member of the Zappos VIP Club. I have no idea what that entails, but I do know that, in that short conversation, I became an even bigger Zappos fan than I was before. ∎

- Align with personal values and inspire pride: One of Patagonia's (Value proposition, 2012) core values, "Environmentalism (serve as a catalyst for personal and corporate action)," helps the company attract and retain the sort of people who share its bone-deep commitment to environmental activism. Beyond that, Patagonia's employees tend to be lovers of the outdoors who use the company's products, which also makes them the company's best sales reps.

Operational and societal relevance

The ideal statement of core values has operational and societal relevance. It is in these two areas that a statement of values often does the most to differentiate your organization from the competition, because a higher degree of specificity is required when talking about relevance (as opposed to feel-good boilerplate):

- **Operational relevance:** One of P&G's operating principles is innovation, which includes this defining statement: "We place great value on big, new consumer innovations" (Purpose, values & principles, n.d.). Guided by this principle, P&G spends almost as much on R&D as all its competitors combined and has tripled its innovation success rate in recent years. Although healthcare costs have consistently been identified as a national crisis for decades, it is the rare hospital or health system that has declared productivity to be a core value. (One exception is Milford Hospital in Milford, Connecticut, whose four core values include "Productivity & Efficiency.")

- **Societal relevance:** The Coca-Cola Company (Workplace culture, 2016) includes diversity as one of its seven core values, including this statement: "Our diversity workplace strategy includes programs to attract, retain, and develop diverse talent; provide support systems for groups with diverse backgrounds; and educate all associates so that we master the skills to achieve sustainable growth." The website goes on to describe specific ways in which the company promotes diversity. To hold to its core value of stewardship, SSM Health requires that each facility have a Preservation of the Earth (POE) committee. The organization has banned plastic bottles and Styrofoam products throughout all its facilities and has recycled millions of pounds of discarded materials.

The Values > Behaviors > Outcomes Continuum

The Values > Behaviors > Outcomes continuum (see Figure 3.1) is a useful construct for evaluating an organization's statement of values. Many of the elements included in such statements are not actually values—they are expected behaviors and desired outcomes. Values are the underlying personal qualities that inspire the behaviors that the organization expects employees to perform in order to achieve the outcomes it desires.

Therefore, when considering a statement of values, it is important to understand which elements are values and which are behaviors and outcomes. Take trust, for example. Stephen M. R. Covey (2006) cogently argues that the absence of trust is like a tax imposed on the organization—it makes everything cost more and take longer than it would be if trust prevailed. So trust is a quality that should be highly valued. But trust itself is not a value. It is an *outcome* that is earned by *behaviors*, including honesty, reliability, and humility. And at a personal level, these behaviors are inspired by a commitment to the *value* of integrity.

It is entirely appropriate to include behaviors and outcomes in a statement of values. Professionalism, courtesy, service, honesty, and reliability are behaviors. Quality, excellence, innovation, growth, and safety are outcomes. Being clear about the outcomes you desire will help you identify the behaviors that are essential to achieve those outcomes. But, to achieve a truly transformative culture, your organization must identify, and your peers and coworkers must embrace, the core values that inspire the behaviors that drive these desired outcomes.

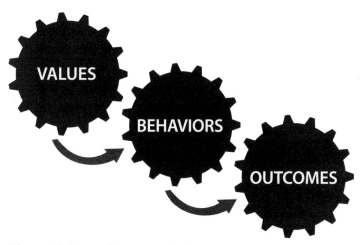

Figure 3.1   *Values inspire behaviors that produce outcomes.*

Source: Cultural Blueprinting Toolkit Workbook

Read your organization's statement of values. Chances are that, like most values statements, it's actually a blend of core values, desired behaviors, and valued outcomes:

- **Values:** Core values are universal and eternal, and they should inspire personal beliefs and behaviors. When the values statement includes *integrity*, what the organization is saying is that it expects employees to be honest and reliable, to treat other people with respect and dignity, and to have the courage to confront people or practices that violate integrity. Corporations do not have integrity—people do (or do not).

- **Behaviors:** Behavioral expectations can be built into job descriptions, performance appraisals, reward systems, and the fabric of organizational culture. They help to define what the organization means by the words used in the statement of values. This can include behaviors that are expected (for example, treating people with respect) and behaviors that will not be tolerated (for example, bullying).

- **Outcomes:** These are, of course, how customers ultimately evaluate the performance of organizations and employees. Excellent customer service, outstanding patient care quality, excellent safety results, and superior financial performance are not values; they are outcomes that derive from professional behaviors.

The core values of Build-A-Bear Workshop are "reach, learn, di-bear-sity, colla-bear-ate, give and cele-bear-ate" ("Why You Should Become a Bear," n.d.). The company carries out its mission—"to bring the Teddy Bear to life"—by striving to embody "warm thoughts about our childhood, about friendship, about trust and comfort, and also about love." Such idiosyncrasies certainly aren't everybody's tastes—it's easy for a cynic to smirk at a value like "di-bear-sity"—but the company's niche culture is self-selecting and self-sustaining. After all, Build-A-Bear has been featured on *Fortune*'s 100 Best Companies to Work For list for 8 straight years.

The Integrated DNA Technologies recruiting web page says: "IDT's Core Values form the foundation of who we are, what we believe, and what we strive to be. They articulate what is expected of us; guiding our relationships and directing our decision making. In our ever evolving business, the Core Values are our constant. Our Core Values define our unique culture, shape our future and ultimately cultivate our success." One of the company's eight core values is "Be yourself—unless you're a jerk" (IDT core values, 2016). In six words, it captures the essential elements of a core value: Be authentic and don't try to impress us by pretending to be someone else; be a team player and treat others with respect; and leave your jerk attitudes in the parking lot. And all in a way that conveys a sense of humor.

Core Value Examples

Here are some of our favorite core values:

- Be yourself, unless you're a jerk. (Integrated DNA Technologies, 2016)

- Give a damn. (Southlake Regional Health Centre, 2012)

- Expect greatness in yourself and inspire it in others. (Clickstop, n.d.)

- Cypress is about winning. We do not tolerate losing. (Cypress Semiconductor, 2011)

- Create fun and a little weirdness. (Zappos, 2010)

- Treat fellow Rackers like Friends and Family. (Rackspace, 2016)

- Our energy and enthusiasm are contagious. We are inspired to make a lasting impact. (Huron, 2016)

- Be fearless. (Playground Inc., 2015)

continues

- Don't take ourselves too seriously; have fun. (AWeber, 2016)

- Create an environment where employees can think big, have fun, and do good. (Warby Parker, n.d.)

- We push for perfection, but never at the expense of progress. (InVision, 2016)

Reviewing and Revising Values

Every 5 years or so the statement of values should be pulled off the wall, literally or figuratively, and subjected to a comprehensive review, reevaluation, and possible revision. This is important because people change, organizations change, and the world changes.

In past years, hospitals have legitimately been criticized for a lack of environmental stewardship. It wasn't that long ago that most hospitals had incinerators out back with which they spewed the residues of all sorts of nasty stuff into the air of surrounding communities. Would including a statement defining your commitment to "stewardship" in your core values encourage your employees to be more responsible about utilizing the hospital's resources, and help the hospital be more aware of its environment footprint? Likewise, if your organization is struggling to recruit and retain younger people, you might need to think about whether work-life balance merits consideration as a core value. You probably wouldn't have seen core values like this in a healthcare organization 20 years ago. Similarly, 20 years ago such concerns as diversity and environmental stewardship weren't seen as being as important as they are today, so you might consider whether your commitment to them should be elevated to the status of core value.

This is not to say that you should blindly follow the latest management fads. Mayo Clinic has maintained the same core values from its inception (Viggiano, Pawlina, Lindor, Olsen, & Cortese, 2007). But if your core values could be taken down from the wall of your organization and tacked up in the lobby of a competitor without anyone thinking it out of place, the exercise will do you good.

In 1943, then-CEO General Robert Wood Johnson, a descendant of the founders of Johnson & Johnson, penned the "J&J Credo," the company's famous statement of duties: to customers first, then employees and communities, and only last to stakeholders. When J&J CEO Jim Burke discovered in 1976 that almost no one in the company knew about the J&J Credo, he launched a company-wide program, called the "Credo Challenge," to train thousands of employees in the company's founding vision and expectations. As part of the program, Burke mandated that every year the company would effectively shut down production for a whole day in order to hold a forum on how to apply the credo in practice.

Then, in 1982, a psychopath added cyanide to Tylenol bottles in supermarkets and pharmacies in the Chicago area, killing seven people who swallowed the poisoned medicine. When the senior executive team of Johnson & Johnson convened an emergency session to discuss the crisis, Burke had already placed copies of the J&J Credo at every team member's seat. Its principles guided their response.

The leadership had conclusively ruled out the possibility of tampering in the manufacturing or distribution processes. Whoever poisoned the bottles had done it at the stores themselves. Burke asked if they were absolutely certain the problem was limited to Chicago. The man responsible nodded, saying that they were 99% certain that was the case. Burke lifted his copy of the Credo and read the first line aloud: "We believe our first responsibility is to the doctors, nurses, and patients, to mothers and fathers and all others who use our products. In meeting their needs, everything we do must be of high quality" (quoted in Ghillyer, 2013, p. 63). If they truly believed that, he said, then 99% was not good enough. Johnson & Johnson pulled Tylenol from retail shelves from coast to coast, offered full refunds, and ran a high-visibility advertising campaign warning people to not use Tylenol.

In the short run, the crisis cost hundreds of millions of dollars in restocking fees alone. Investors panicked, and J&J's stock price dropped 20%. And as it turned out, the problem was in fact limited to Chicago. In the long run, though, the company's courage to do the right thing regardless of the cost earned it unparalleled trust and goodwill. "I think the answers come down from the value system," Burke said in the aftermath of the crisis. "What's right works. It really does. The cynics will tell you it doesn't, but they're wrong" (quoted in Melé, 2009, p. 19).

Burke's prediction was proven out in subsequent years as billions of dollars in goodwill accrued to the J&J balance sheet as a result of the trust the company had earned. When it faced severe financial challenges in the immediate aftermath of the tragedy, one group of employees commissioned custom T-shirts that read, "We're coming back." Upon learning who would wear the T-shirts, the CEO of the garment company that had produced them waived the charge.

Unfortunately, in subsequent years J&J has strayed from its Credo and has paid a substantial price in both monetary fines and tarnished reputation for doing so, culminating in a 15-part investigation of the company's suspect ethics and dubious practices published by the Huffington Post under the title "America's Most Admired Law Breaker" (Brill, 2015).

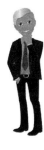

A Note from Joe

My wife, Sally, has an enlarged ascending aorta. We had an appointment for her to see a cardiac surgeon at the Mayo Clinic on the very day that the hospital displaced Johns Hopkins as number one in *U.S. News & World Report*'s rankings of American hospitals. The visit started with a 1-hour meeting with a nurse practitioner. She was thoroughly prepared for the session, answered every question (even my dumb questions) with the utmost respect, and for that hour made us feel like we were the only people in the building. When we had thoroughly exhausted our questions, she told us that she would see whether the surgeon could see us sooner than our scheduled appointment 2 hours hence, because we had a long drive home.

My daughter was, at the time, working on a PhD in neurobiology research (and has since graduated). She had searched for information about this surgeon online beforehand and reported that he was "a rock star" in the medical community, so we didn't get our hopes up that he would be able to rearrange his schedule. But he arrived 10 minutes later and then spent the next 45 minutes making us feel like we were the only people in the building. By the time we left the cardiac surgery clinic and reached the front door, three different people, including a housekeeper and someone pushing a food cart, stopped to ask whether we needed help.

I'm sure there are fine surgeons in hospitals that are closer and more convenient to see than at Mayo Clinic, but when the time comes for Sally to have her surgery, that is where we will go. I know I can trust a hospital when everyone from the guy pushing a food cart to the world-renowned cardiac surgeon is thinking and acting like they own the place. ■

Questions to Ask About Your Organization's Core Values

Think of your core values as the final answers to a vast series of implicit questions. What is the essence of what you do? What matters most to you, and to the people you serve? When things go wrong, how do you respond? The list is endless. But here are a few crucial questions to ask about any and every statement of values after it's finished. If you can't answer them to your own satisfaction, maybe the statement of values isn't as finished as you thought.

Why were our values chosen and others left out? Because there are literally hundreds of ways to phrase these values, this is an important process for establishing organizational identity.

Do these values reflect who we are as an organization today and who we want to be in the future? Core values should be both descriptive and aspirational. They must reflect what your organization is today and what makes it unique, and also inspire employees to continuously raise the bar for the future.

Are our organization's values operationally relevant? In addition to warm-and-fuzzy concepts like compassion and integrity, look to elevate essential operating parameters, such as productivity and loyalty, to the status of being core values.

Are our organization's values socially relevant? Make sure the values properly reflect the societal responsibility for the environment, for the underserved, and for public health and mental health.

Would we keep these values if our organization were punished for following them? There is often a price to be paid for acting on values—for example, reporting a Medicare violation that could result in substantial fines. They are not truly core values unless leaders are willing to pay that price.

Are our organization's values worded in such a way that they inspire employees to take ownership for them because they resonate with their own personal values? Many organizational values statements sound more like legalistic boilerplate than something that is meant to touch the hearts of the people who work there.

If someone from another organization copied our statement of values verbatim and posted it in their organization's lobby, would anyone know that it had been lifted? A generic values statement that does not differentiate your organization from competitors represents a missed opportunity, both for polishing your reputation in the community and for attracting the right kind of people to apply for jobs.

How would a space alien see our organization's values actually being reflected (or not) in the attitudes and behaviors of our employees? A statement of values that is tacked up on the wall but not reflected in actual employee attitudes and behaviors is worse than no statement of values at all.

When should we next revisit and, if appropriate, revise our statement of core values? In today's fast-changing healthcare environment, it makes sense to periodically review your statement of values in light of societal, technological, and generational changes that have occurred since it was first created.

The Interaction of Personal and Organizational Values

As of this writing (in 2016), Emily Wynn is the interim associate chief nursing officer at University of Iowa Hospitals and Clinics. In job interviews and in performance reviews, she covers both competence goals and character goals. Emily says that a competence goal might be to achieve a certain level of certification, and a character goal might be to learn how to be more open to constructive feedback from peers. While employees are generally clear about their competence goals, she says, they tend to struggle when asked about character goals. And though it is relatively easy to manage performance expectations that require skills and competence, it is much more difficult to manage behavioral expectations that are based on character.

At Park Ridge Health, a member of Adventist Health System in Hendersonville, North Carolina, chief nursing officer Craig Lindsey explains to all job applicants that the company's culture is based on the Christian faith and that staff and physicians are encouraged to pray with patients or to connect them with hospital chaplains. When one otherwise highly qualified physician candidate said in an interview that he didn't care what patients believed as long as they didn't interfere with his practice of medicine, the hospital staff realized that he would not be a good fit and did not offer him a position.

When Sidra Medical and Research Center, a magnificent healthcare and educational facility in Doha, Qatar, was built, its leadership team commissioned Values Coach to help them create a cultural blueprint for its Invisible Architecture to ensure that both the employee and patient experience would

"Values are fundamentally about interpersonal relationships or social architecture or culture. I think of values in an organization as having two closely interrelated aspects: organizational values and personal values."

–James A. Autry,
The Servant Leader

mirror the beautiful physical facilities. One core value that is defined in the Sidra behavioral framework is innovation. This value is supported by a statement outlining a philosophy of freedom to innovate, welcoming new ideas and encouraging creativity, supporting talent, creating confidence, and celebrating success. The framework then establishes these principles to provide a guide for personal attitudes and behaviors:

- Displays curiosity and creativity and evaluates risk-taking to explore new ideas
- Takes the initiative to go beyond assigned responsibilities and goals within the scope of practice
- Offers and encourages ideas and actions that will benefit Sidra, our patients and families, staff, and Qatar
- Embraces improvements and changes to processes as opportunities for learning and growth that contribute to a world-class healthcare organization
- Positively engages colleagues across Sidra to harness and build on employee experience and best practices
- Gives credit to others and recognizes and celebrates wins

Why Many Healthcare Values Statements Don't Work

We have had the opportunity to review hundreds of organizational values statements, including many from healthcare organizations. This section describes the most common problems in the values statements of healthcare organizations.

Inauthenticity

If your values statement could be moved from your wall and posted in the lobby of a competitor without anyone taking notice, you have not defined a set of core values that is authentic to your organization. If you see a values statement that includes "Create fun and a little weirdness" anywhere other than Zappos, you'll know it's a knockoff. Defining "Give a damn" as a core value is how Southlake Regional Health Centre in Toronto tells employees and prospective employees that they are expected to think and act like owners. When it comes to authenticity, the style is just as important as the sentiment.

Minimal expectations

Despite the highfalutin language, many values statements actually set a low bar for performance expectations. Of course, your organization expects integrity and excellent performance from employees—so does the cupcake shop downtown. And while we certainly hope that your caregivers live out the value of being empathetic, we also know that patrons expect empathy from their barbers and bartenders.

One core value at Cypress Semiconductor is this: "Cypress is about winning. We do not tolerate losing." Another is, "We make our numbers" (Who we are, 2011). Cypress Semiconductor did not create a feel-good, touchy-feely set of values; its statement is precisely focused on the operational requirements for creating "The Marine Corps of Silicon Valley" culture that defines the company. You might not like the tough language, but the intention is crystal-clear. And that clarity is one reason why Cypress—whose CEO wrote the book *No Excuses Management*—almost never makes hiring mistakes.

Boilerplate

All too often, values statements read as though they were written by a lawyer or, worse, a committee of public relations interns. The declarations are formulaic; the exhortations, predictable. There's no *life* in the words. Their boilerplate wording describes characteristics that you think people expect of you rather than say something important about who you really are. If your values look like they were created by a *Dilbert Core Values Statement Generator*, they are probably doing little to create competitive differentiation, to inspire pride among your employees, or to earn the loyalty of patients.

Here's a simple test to see whether your statement of values fails that test: Imagine a typical employee going home and sharing those values with a child who is considering multiple possibilities for a first job. If the child's eyes glaze over, you are probably missing a great opportunity to connect people from a younger generation with the values that define who you are, what you stand for, and what you won't stand for. When it comes to attracting the bright young superstars of the future, no matter what industry you happen to be in, you are competing against the likes of Google, HubSpot, Zappos, and other dynamic organizations that take values and culture seriously—and that have been remarkably successful at recruiting bright young people for entry-level jobs.

Acronyms

An acronym can be a useful memory aid for a statement of values, but it can also suck the life out of that statement by turning it into something that is bland and generic. Acronyms can also, quite inadvertently, establish a low standard of expectations. ICARE is a popular one; without even knowing the identity of the organization, it's easy to guess which values have been force-fitted into the ICARE formula: Integrity, Compassion, Accountability, Respect, and Excellence are typical in healthcare organizations (Tye, 2015). (See the sidebar for similar real-world examples.) These are admirable values to claim, but they do little to distinguish your organization from any other that claims the same or similar values. For that matter, most people expect such ICARE values from the local grocery store.

The Unbearable Sameness of ICARE

Many organizations use the ICARE acronym to represent their core values. There's nothing inherently wrong with ICARE, and there's certainly nothing wrong with caring. But if your values are the same, and said the same way, as everybody else's, how valuable are they? Instead of offering a catchy way to remember values, ICARE statements invariably come off as flat and uninspiring. Here are a few examples:

- **Veterans Health Administration:** Integrity, Commitment, Advocacy, Respect, and Excellence

- **Houston Methodist:** Integrity, Compassion, Accountability, Respect, and Excellence

- **University of Rochester Medical Center:** Integrity, Compassion, Accountability, Respect, and Excellence

- **Mercy Medical Center (more than one):** Integrity, Compassion, Accountability, Respect, and Excellence

- **Goodwill Industries:** Integrity, Collaboration, Attitude, Respect, and Explore

- **Boys & Girls Club of America:** Integrity, Collaboration, Accountability, Respect, and Excellence

- **Supplemental Healthcare:** Integrity, Candor, Accountability, Respect, and Excellence

- **McKesson Corporation:** Integrity, Customer-First, Accountability, Respect, and Excellence

When it comes to acronyms, the most important question is, which came first—the values or the letters? If the organization has defined its true core values and, quite by coincidence, they happen to lend themselves to an easy-to-remember acronym, that can be a beautiful thing. On the other hand, if the organization has forced an assortment of words into a pre-determined acronym, employees might remember the words without ever truly embracing the underlying commitments.

The seven core values of the United States Army are represented by the acronym LDRSHIP (The Army values, 2016). Though this acronym is a useful memory aid, it is clearly a serendipitous case of the values' first letters aligning and not the values having been force-fitted into a pre-conceived acronym (as often appears to be the case with the ICARE acronym). The U.S. Army values are:

Loyalty: Bear true faith and allegiance to the U.S. Constitution, the Army, your unit, and other soldiers.

Duty: Fulfill your obligations.

Respect: Treat people as they should be treated.

Selfless service: Put the welfare of the nation, the Army, and your subordinates before your own.

Honor: Live up to all Army values.

Integrity: Do what's right, legally and morally.

Personal courage: Face fear, danger, or adversity (physical or moral).

One example of an effective values statement acronym is that of Edward-Elmhurst Health, a three-hospital healthcare system in Illinois. It uses the acronym DRIVEN for the core values of Determination, Respect, Integrity, Vision, Excellence, and Nurturing. The tagline on its website is "We are healthy driven. We believe in keeping your health moving forward as far down the road as humanly possible" (Healthy driven, 2016). But what really makes it work is the web strategy developed by MedTouch (a company that helps hospitals develop and implement digital and web strategies; www.medtouch.com). The hospital recruited professional racecar driver Danica Patrick to serve as its ambassador, with the *Healthy Driven with Danica*

Patrick monthly blog on healthful lifestyle choices. Its health risk assessment web page features a picture of Patrick saying that it's "Like an engine check, for people." By weaving the Healthy Driven theme through multiple different sections of the website, the values seem more real—and, dare we say, more driven.

Lack of relevance

Ask any frontline nurse what the CEO of the company values more highly: compassion or productivity. Chances are great that the answer will be *productivity*. But it is the rare healthcare organization that has elevated productivity to the level of a core value (which in today's world, it should be). Ironically, the first person ever to measure hospital productivity was Florence Nightingale, who more than any other individual created a blueprint for the modern hospital as we know it. Nightingale was the first healthcare executive ever to calculate cost per patient day, which to this day is a core measure of hospital productivity. She intuitively understood the relationship between productivity and the organization's ability to provide compassionate care that is reflected in the aphorism "no margin, no mission."

Not featured in recruiting

An organization that has, and more importantly, acts in accordance with, a strong set of core values has an inherent advantage in recruiting against competitors who are more muddled about their values. When a culture's values are unclear, the culture is typically incoherent; it just *feels off*. Securely values-based companies "will naturally attract the right employees and repel the wrong ones. This makes recruiting exponentially easier and more effective, and it drastically reduces turnover" (Lencioni, 2012, p. 91). If you look at recruitment web pages for any of the companies on the *Fortune* magazine roster of the 100 Best Companies to Work For, the first thing you are likely to see is a description of that organization's values and culture. Check out the Careers page of your own organization. If the first thing you see is a listing of open positions and an online application form, you are missing a great opportunity to attract employees who resonate with your core values (and to screen out people who don't).

Brass plaques

Many organizational values statements are enshrined, at least metaphorically and often literally, in a brass plaque on the wall. Chances are good that you put more time and money into the design of a promotional flyer than you do the visual presentation of the most important document in your organization: your statement of core values. A great graphical design is a way of placing values front and center. Jarrard, a healthcare PR firm in Brentwood, Tennessee, has a beautiful display in the main lobby of its office featuring a representative icon for each of the company's 11 core values. If the graphical presentation of your core values wouldn't make an attractive billboard, like the one for Tucson Medical Center, shown in Figure 3.2, send your graphic designer back to the drawing boards.

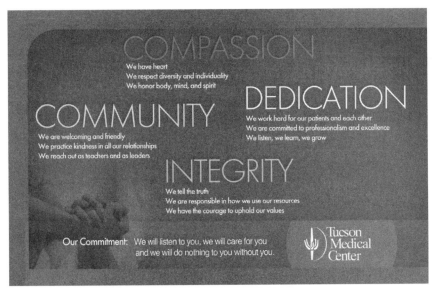

Figure 3.2 *Give your core values an attractive design.*

Read your own organization's statement of values and compare it against these common problems. Then ask yourself (or your CEO) whether it is time to take the brass plaque off the wall and reconsider the values statement itself or the way it is presented.

The Great Wyoming Values and Culture Challenge

In 2013, Values Coach worked with Memorial Hospital of Converse County in eastern Wyoming and Star Valley Medical Center in western Wyoming on The Great Wyoming Values and Culture Challenge. The purpose of this initiative was to utilize a creative approach to help each organization spark a cultural transformation in a way that gave it more the feel of a cross-state sports rivalry than a management program. An independent review panel of nationally recognized authorities on healthcare was established to review the work of each organization. Specific goals included:

- Challenge employees at each hospital to hold themselves and each other to a higher standard of behavior by committing to a shared set of personal values and doing so in a way that is fun and inspiring, and with a lasting impact on the lives of employees and their loved ones.

- Challenge each hospital's leadership team to establish a process for creating a cultural blueprint for its Invisible Architecture to complement the one it has for its bricks-and-mortar buildings and a culture plan to complement its current strategic plan.

- Spark a cultural transformation in each organization that fosters a more positive and productive workplace, enhances employee engagement and patient satisfaction, and builds each hospital's reputation for being a great place to work.

- Reach out from the platform of the hospital to engage the broader community in a dialogue about, and commitment to, values—beginning with the families of employees.

- Implement processes, routines, rituals, and habits that ensure a sustained impact on both the organization and the community.

- Develop and implement creative and innovative ideas that can be shared with other hospitals and communities across the country, including by way of publications (white papers, journal articles, etc.).

- Have fun while making a difference in people's lives.

As part of the process, each hospital created a new statement of core values. Taking different approaches to developing these statements let them come up with quite different statements that reflected, in many ways, the personalities of the organizations and their communities.

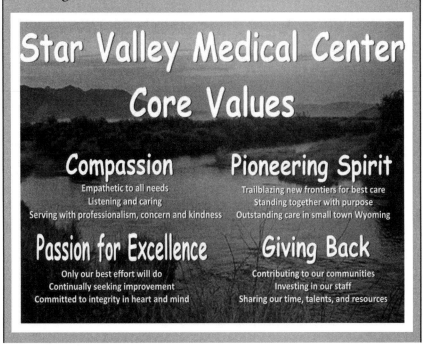

"Invisible Architecture"

Memorial Hospital of Converse County is more than a place, it is a culture, built upon our seven essential values. These values, as described by America's Values Coach, Joe Tye, are our organization's Invisible architecture, the unseen support of our hospital's culture. They are what define us, molding the behavioral standards we choose most important as an organization.

Integrity

We hold ourselves accountable to the highest ethical and performance standards, demonstrating honesty, professionalism and sincerity. Therefore ...

- I will always speak honestly & tactfully
- I will talk with, and not about, others
- I will do what I say and say what I do
- I will treat everyone with dignity
- I will own and work to correct my mistakes

Respect

We believe respect for one's self and for others is the foundation of honor and the basis of integrity. Such respect is essential for nurturing the innovative spirit of our hospital. Therefore ...

- I will seek to make all people feel valued & appreciated
- I will be professional, courteous, honest & thoughtful in all my interactions
- I will protect confidentiality – knowing my audience
- I will protect others privacy – knocking before entering

Ownership

We believe in taking ownership for ones responsibilities and goals. As owners we recognize it is our responsibility to do what is right for our patients, our hospital and our coworkers. We understand each of us plays a critical role in fulfilling our mission. Therefore ...

- I will not say, "It's not my job" or "we are short-staffed"
- I am available to assist, encourage and help others
- I will be a good steward of all resources
- I will take responsibility for my actions and behavior
- I will think "team," sharing successes & failures together

Patient-Centered

We provide care that is respectful of and responsive to individual patient preferences, needs, and values. We will remember that people are our reason for our being here, not an interruption of our work. Therefore ...

- I will actively "see" and "listen to" others
- I will rush to meet their needs, exceeding their expectations
- I will genuinely care for others as I want to be treated
- I will respect others dignity and privacy
- When we fail to meet expectations, I will acknowledge, apologize, and make amends

Compassion

We recognize every person as a whole human being with different needs that must be met through listening, empathizing and nurturing. Therefore ...

- I will be hospitable, anticipating others needs
- I will listen attentively and act on what I hear
- I will strive to relieve fears and anxieties
- I will advocate for my patients and co-workers
- I will use AIDET:
    Acknowledge, Introduce, Duration, Explanation, Thank you

Competency

We are dedicated to employing, training, and providing staff with the appropriate tools needed to respond to the unique needs of our patients, our coworkers, and our community. Therefore ...

- I will make sure that I am well-trained in all aspects of my job
- If I do not know what to do or how to do something I will ask
- I will always practice safety, and use best practices with confidence
- I will seek to continually improve my job skills and people skills
- I will provide private, constructive feedback for inappropriate behaviors
    When interviewing, I will strive to hire only the best

Joy

We believe employees who enjoy their role within the organization and their relationships with one another create a healthy environment for all. We look for both fun and humor, when appropriate, in our daily work. Therefore ...

- I will make an honest effort to always be positive
- I will look for the best in people and situations
- I will smile while greeting everyone – whether in person or on the phone
- I will seek to see the positive in stressful situations
- I will seek to lift the spirits of all around me

MEMORIAL HOSPITAL
of Converse County
Advanced Medicine. Hometown Care.

Values, Culture, and Adversity

In August of 2005, HCA, also known as Hospital Corporation of America, was faced with a severe crisis as Hurricane Katrina hammered the New Orleans area, where HCA has several hospitals, including Tulane University Hospital. HCA employees went to heroic lengths to save lives during the darkest days of the flood and in the following months to help the thousands of people whose lives had been disrupted (Carey, 2006). HCA's commitment was not limited to its own facilities—HCA employees were also instrumental in evacuating and accommodating patients and employees from nearby Charity Hospital.

In an interview for this book, a senior HCA executive told us that the company's response to Hurricane Katrina and the subsequent floods was "the defining moment in HCA's history." Then-CEO Jack Bovender received thousands of emails from HCA employees. This single sentence excerpt captures the spirit of all of the others: "I want to say that in 25 years of being in healthcare, never have I been so proud to be affiliated with an employer as I am at this moment" (Carey, 2006, p. 157).

One of the reasons HCA's leadership acted almost instinctively to "do the right thing now and ask about the cost later" is that the company's values and culture had been severely tested, and subsequently reshaped, by a previous crisis. In 1993, HCA merged with another hospital operations company, Columbia, to form Columbia/HCA. The company grew fast—much too fast—and it fell apart in 1997 amid a federal corruption investigation. The board ousted CEO Rick Scott and brought back HCA cofounder Dr. Thomas Frist Jr. to turn the company around. "Perhaps the most critical piece of the 12-point plan" created by Dr. Frist in collaboration with Bovender, "was fostering a values-based culture" (Rodengen, 2003, p. 107).

A toxic culture fixated on growth regardless of the cost led to the collapse of Columbia/HCA. That catastrophe led, in turn, to the introspection and commitment that forged the culture of a company that crafted a textbook response during Katrina and that continues to be respected and recognized for its commitment to integrity.

When (in most cases it is *when* and not *if)* you find your organization in a crisis, will your values and culture help you rise to the occasion or will you sink in the flood? And what are the implications of your answer for the priorities you will set for the rest of this week?

Words on a Wall: The Downside of Losing Sight of Your Values

The most catastrophic failures in business, and in personal life, do not come from failed strategies—they come from a failure of values. In fact, a good way to judge an organization's health is to measure its observable behavior against its declared values, as shown in a long line of corporate crash-and-burn stories. And the same can be said for the individual, as reflected in the rapid descent of Lance Armstrong from one of the most admired to one of the most despised people on the planet.

> **"**
>
> If we lose sight of our vision and bury our values, then we have lost our soul.
>
> —David Whyte,
> *The Heart Aroused:
> Poetry and the Preservation
> of the Soul in Corporate
> America*
>
> **"**

According to Jim Collins (2009, p. 100), you can diagnose an organization in Stage 4 decline (the stage just before irrelevance and oblivion set in) based on the following symptoms: "People cannot easily articulate what the company stands for, core values have eroded to the point of irrelevance, the organization has become 'just another place to work,' a place to get a pay-check, and people lose faith in their ability to triumph and prevail."

Enron has become shorthand for valueless leadership and corporate corruption. Enron's bankruptcy stood as the largest in U.S. history—until the next year, when telecom darling WorldCom dissolved after three of its employees discovered evidence that $3.8 billion was missing in the organization's cooked books. Embezzlement was so rife at multinational behemoth Tyco International that two of its key executives were sentenced to up to 25 years in prison.

The Acid Test of Living Your Values

According to workplace culture expert Robert Richman, the true test of whether an organization is serious about val-ues "all comes down to this: Are you willing to fire some-one who does not fit the values, despite their performance?" (2015, p. 62).

In early 2009, Values Coach worked with the leadership team of Tucson Medical Center—the largest independent hospital in Tucson, Arizona—to create a statement of values that was more genuine and meaningful than the boilerplate statement that, up to that point, almost no one even knew existed. The hospital had experienced a period of consider-able uncertainty and anxiety while the board was engaged in a due-diligence process that might have resulted in sale of the facility. Once the decision was made to remain independent, CEO Judy Rich wanted to reconnect people with core values that truly would define who they are, what they stand for, and what they won't stand for.

Over a period of months, Joe researched the history of the hospital, interviewed several hundred people in individual and focus group settings, and conducted all-employee town meetings. He then worked with Judy and her executive team to finalize a statement featuring four "pillar" values, each supported by three statements of commitment (refer to Figure 3-2). Not coincidentally, within 9 months of that values statement being adopted by the board, overall patient satisfaction (HCAHPS) scores went up by 10 points.

Shortly after the Tucson Medical Center's values had been formally approved by the board, a hospital executive saw a bumper sticker on a car in the employee parking lot that read, "I'm a nurse—my job is to save your ass, not to kiss it." The toxic attitude reflected in that bumper sticker was clearly in conflict with the medical center's core values. It was discovered that the nurse who owned the car had already had multiple warnings about attitude problems. The nurse was called in and told she had a choice to make: She could have the bumper sticker, or she could have an employee parking sticker on her windshield. When she refused to remove the bumper sticker, her employment was terminated.

Summary

A statement of core values is one of the most important documents in your organization. A great statement of values can create a significant competitive advantage for positioning your organization in the marketplace in recruiting for talent. It should define who you are, what you stand for, and what you won't stand for and should have both operational and societal relevance. It is important to periodically review, and when appropriate revise, your statement of values.

Chapter Questions

- Do the people who work in your organization know its core values by heart (not just by rote memory, but *by heart*)? Are your values prominently featured on your website; included in recruiting, new employee orientation, and performance appraisal; and serving as a source of pride for employees?

- Do your values stand out and differentiate your organization, or would they not seem out of place on the wall of a competitor? Are employees who are parents proud to share your organizational values with their children?

- When is the last time your organization's statement of values was reevaluated? Should that happen now, and if so, what would be the best process for doing it?

- Does your leadership team reflect your values in their actual behavior, and do they have the courage to expect that others will as well?

References

Autry, J. A. (2001). *The servant leader: How to build a creative team, develop great morale, and improve bottom-line performance.* Roseville, CA: Prima Pub.

AWeber. (2016). Core values: Our blueprint for success. Retrieved from https://blog.aweber.com/email-marketing/core-values-our-blueprint-for-success.htm

Brill, S. (2015). America's most admired lawbreaker. The Huffington Post Highline. Retrieved from http://highline.huffingtonpost.com/miracleindustry/americas-most-admired-lawbreaker/chapter-1.html

Build-A-Bear. (n.d.). Why you should become a bear. Retrieved from https://careers.buildabear.com/AboutUs.aspx

Carey, B. (2006). *Leave no one behind: Hurricane Katrina and the rescue of Tulane Hospital.* Nashville, TN: Clearbrook Press.

Clickstop. (n.d.). Expect greatness in yourself and inspire it in others. Retrieved from http://clickstop.com/about-us/culture/clickstop-core-values/expect-greatness-in-yourself-and-inspire-it-in-others/

Coca-Cola Company. (2016). Workplace culture. Retrieved from http://www.coca-colacompany.com/our-company/diversity/workplace-culture

Collins, J. C. (2009). *How the mighty fall: And why some companies never give in*. New York, NY: HarperCollins.

Covey, S. M. R. (2006). *The speed of trust: Why trust is the ultimate determinant of success or failure in your relationships, career and life*. London, England: Simon & Schuster.

Cypress Semiconductor Corporation. (2011). Who we are. Retrieved from http://www.cypress.com/about-cypress

Edward-Elmhurst Health. (2016). Healthy driven. Retrieved from https://www.eehealth.org/healthy-driven

Ghillyer, A. W. (2013). *Business ethics now*. New York, NY: McGraw-Hill Education.

Griffin Hospital. (n.d.). Mission & values. Retrieved from http://www.griffinhealth.org/about/griffin-health/mission-values

Hsieh, T. (2010). *Delivering happiness: A path to profits, passion, and purpose*. New York, NY: Business Plus.

Huron. (2016). About us. Retrieved from https://www.huronconsultinggroup.com/company/about-us

Integrated DNA Technologies. (2016). IDT core values. Retrieved from www.idtdna.com/pages/home/about-us/core-values

InVision. (2016). Good design is good for business. Retrieved from https://www.invisionapp.com/company

Lencioni, P. (2012). *The advantage: Why organizational health trumps everything else in business*. San Francisco, CA: Jossey-Bass.

Melé, D. (2009). *Business ethics in action: Seeking human excellence in organizations*. Basingstoke, England: Palgrave Macmillan.

Milford Hospital. (2010). Mission. Retrieved from http://www.milfordhospital.org/about/mission/

Modern Survey. (2013). State of engagement: Unveiling Modern Survey's latest U.S. employee research. Retrieved from https://www.hr.com/en?t=/network/event/attachment.supply&fileID=1397754242330

Patagonia. (2012). Value proposition. Retrieved from https://patagoniacompany.wordpress.com/2012/05/10/value-proposition/

Peters, T. J., & Waterman, R. H. (1982). *In search of excellence: Lessons from America's best-run companies*. New York, NY: Harper & Row.

Playground, Inc. (2015). We are a digital creative agency. Retrieved from http://playgroundinc.com/

Procter & Gamble. (2016). Purpose, values & principles. Retrieved from https://us.pg.com/who-we-are/our-approach/purpose-values-principles

Rackspace. (2016). What's at the core of Rackspace core values? Retrieved from http://blog.rackspace.com/whats-core-rackspace-core-values

Richman, R. (2015). The culture blueprint: A guide to building the high-performance workplace. Creative Commons.

Rodengen, J. L. (2003). *The legend of HCA: Hospital Corporation of America*. Fort Lauderdale, FL: Write Stuff Enterprises.

Ryan, M. J. (2007). On becoming exceptional: SSM Health Care's journey to Baldrige and beyond. Milwaukee, WI: ASQ Quality Press.

Southlake Regional Health Centre. (2012). Our core commitments. Retrieved from http://www.southlakeregional.org/Default.aspx?cid=665&lang=1

Sullivan, G. R., & Harper, M. V. (1996). *Hope is not a method: What business leaders can learn from America's Army.* New York, NY: Times Business.

U.S. Army. (2016). The Army values. Retrieved from https://www.army.mil/values

Viggiano, T. R., Pawlina, W., Lindor, K. D., Olsen, K. D., & Cortese, D. A. (2007). Putting the needs of the patient first: Mayo Clinic's core value, institutional culture, and professionalism covenant. *Academic Medicine, 82*(11), 1089-1093.

Warby Parker. (n.d.). We have a couple of ground rules at Warby Parker. Retrieved from https://www.warbyparker.com/culture

Whyte, D. (1994). *The heart aroused: Poetry and the preservation of the soul in corporate America.* New York, NY: Currency Doubleday.

Zappos. (n.d.). About Zappos culture. Retrieved from http://www.zappos.com/core-values

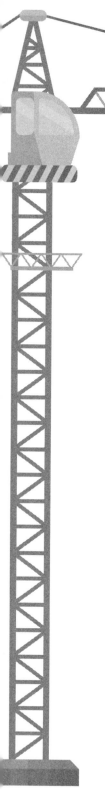

"

Culture influences how we deliver care,
how we interrelate with our colleagues,
and how we treat our patients.

"

—Peter Pronovost,
Safe Patients, Smart Hospitals

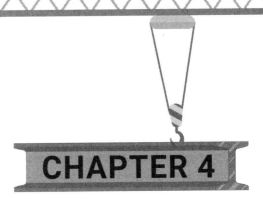

CHAPTER 4

The Superstructure of Organizational Culture

Chapter Goals

- Explain why a great culture is vitally important for both the employee and the patient experience and is a non-negotiable element of being recognized as being a great place to work.
- Share 10 reasons why Peter Drucker is right that culture eats strategy for lunch, illustrating each one with real-world examples.
- Describe the concept of the culture code that originated in Silicon Valley, the Values Coach 4-P model for creating a cultural blueprint, and ways that stories (including 6-word stories) can shape culture.
- Explain that culture does not change unless and until people change, because culture is an organizational reflection of the collective attitudes and behaviors of the people who work there.

It's an old story, but a good one: Two young fish are swimming along, minding their business, when they come upon an adult fish passing the other way. The adult says, "Morning, boys. How's the water?" The two youths swim on until, finally, one looks at the other and asks, "What the hell is water?" The moral is that it is possible to be immersed in something but still be oblivious to it, even unaware of its existence. Explaining water to a fish is like explaining air to a child—it is everywhere, but it is invisible; you can feel it, but you can't touch it; and, most importantly, you can't live without it.

If you stand on a street corner in any major American city wearing a pair of men's underpants on your head like a hat, people will think you're weird. There's no law against it, and nobody can quite explain why you shouldn't do it, but everybody will know it's *just weird*. That's culture in action. If someone is doing push-ups in an airport waiting area when everyone else is watching television, people around him will think he's the one who's weird. That, too, is culture in action. For better or worse (for better and worse!), culture influences people's perceptions of practically everything.

Culture is the umbrella term for every part of the environment that isn't bolted down or paved over: rules and regulations, traditions and customs, habits and routines, shared assumptions and superstitions—even the arts and sciences. It encompasses the *what* and the *how* of what people do, say, and believe. The mind-bending hugeness of this idea leads some people, even some leaders, to dismiss culture as a concept that's too touchy-feely and fuzzy to be important for management to take seriously. They say culture is impossible to change, and so it is too much trouble to bother thinking about.

But culture can change. Not only that—it *will* change, inevitably, as its people change. People and culture are one and the same. What's more, the concrete consequences of culture, and culture change, are immediate and often decisive. The question is whether culture change is conscious and strategic or allowed to happen in an unplanned and haphazard manner.

Some cultures are dreary and depressing, but the best are exhilarating and inspiring. It's because of that culture that the June 10, 2013, cover of *Bloomberg Businessweek* declared Costco "The Cheapest, Happiest Company in The World," and profiled the company's ecstatic employees (Stone). Costco's rule-bound rival Walmart has never been accused of having ecstatic employees; rather, there have been stories of Walmart employees striking over wages and working conditions, and even of the company unlawfully firing picketing employees (Paglieri, 2016). You can make people salute, but you can't make them laugh. Walmart and Costco sell the same sorts of products to the same market segments and with nearly identical pricing strategies, but the experience of being an employee or a customer could not be more different. People pay for the privilege of shopping at Costco by purchasing a membership; most people who shop at Walmart do so because its products are cheap and ubiquitous, not because of loyalty or emotional commitment.

Wall Street and Silicon Valley have a lot in common, but they feel quite different. The same could be said about the Army and the Navy, a public high school and a private academy, or a county jail and a maximum security federal prison. Cultural differences don't have to be extreme to be extremely significant.

In many organizations, former IBM CEO Lou Gerstner (2002) noted, "[M]ost of the really important rules aren't written down anywhere." It's easy, on the other hand, to figure out "what the culture encourages and discourages, rewards and punishes. Is it a culture that rewards individual achievement or team play? Does it value risk taking or consensus building?" (p. 182). Healthcare organizations invite a range of similar, but field-specific, questions. Does the culture encourage workers to admit when they make mistakes, or do they play the shame-and-blame game of pointing fingers and covering for themselves? Does it reward people for taking initiative, or suggest that going the extra mile isn't worth the trouble? Does it tolerate cruelty and intimidation, or do people confront bullying and mean-spirited gossip when they arise?

Culture is the personality and character of the organization. It is shaped by the collective attitudes and actions of the people who make it up. But in most healthcare organizations, there is not one single culture, and probably never will be. Rather, a healthcare organization is like a patchwork quilt of subcultures, including nursing, pharmacy, environmental services, the business office, and the medical staff. These subcultures often have sub-subcultures—within nursing alone, there are significant differences between medical-surgical, critical care, perioperative, emergency, and long-term care. Different cultures can even exist within one unit, depending on staffing and timing (as anyone who has worked both day and night shifts can attest).

The fact that every culture is dynamic and always in a certain amount of flux presents challenges, but it is ultimately a blessing. For a culture to be totally unified, every person in it would have to be exactly the same, to behave the same way and believe the same things. There's nothing more boring (with the possible exception of a boilerplate values statement). Diversity is crucial, but so is commonality. A shared purpose and shared values are crucial to making a culture into a community—or, better still, a culture of ownership.

The question is whether your culture is beautiful and functional or ugly and dysfunctional (or worse yet that it takes the fun out of dysfunctional!). Think of the diverse array of organizational subcultures as sections in a patchwork quilt: The individual pieces might look quite different from each other, but when they are stitched together, the whole is greater (and more useful) than the sum of its parts. It's the same with a great organizational culture: It embraces multiple subcultures while providing a consistent, overarching pattern that coordinates each unit with the whole. Autonomy and adaptability are indispensable in all levels of professional healthcare, but cultural fragmentation can promote debilitating behaviors: power struggles, infighting, incompatible practices, bullying, gossiping, and, in extreme cases, sabotage.

The Best Cultures at Work

Most people in business have heard of the Fortune 500, *Fortune* magazine's annual ranking of the largest corporations in the United States by total revenue. The list is perennially topped by the titans of industry, commerce, and finance: big oil, big banks, big-box stores, and utilities powerhouses. But few of the companies on the Fortune 500 make it onto *Fortune*'s other—and in some ways, more important—list: 100 Best Companies to Work For. There are now many "best places to work" lists, but the Fortune 100 was the first and is still the gold standard.

Every year, *Fortune* teams up with the Great Place to Work Institute to compile this list based on two factors:

- *Fortune* conducts the most wide-ranging employee survey in corporate America, the Trust Index Employee Survey, which quantifies "employees' attitudes about management's credibility, overall job satisfaction, and camaraderie" (2016).
- *Fortune* conducts a detailed "culture audit" of each organization's workplace climate and employee treatment, including pay and benefits, formal recognition, community outreach opportunities, staff diversity, hiring and training practices, and the efficiency and efficacy of internal communications.

As you would expect, the best companies offer outstanding benefits, generous compensation packages, and flexible schedules. But, just as crucially, these companies offer their employees a constellation of less tangible benefits as well: a sense of pride, of mission, and of contribution to the community. Work at these companies is not just work—it is work with a purpose, a meaningful and enriching part of a life well lived, rather than a distraction or an unfortunate but necessary sacrifice. What the list really measures is employee satisfaction. Happiness. Joy. The pleasure and pride of going to work every day for a company that values and honors the work as well as the worker.

As part of the survey process, *Fortune* asks companies what kinds of qualities they look for in prospective employees—not professional skills or credentials (those are a given), but rather characteristics, personality traits, and habits. If you look at the responses of the dozen hospitals and/or health systems featured on *Fortune*'s list, you'll notice something: Each one puts a huge emphasis on cultural fit and the core values *shared between* the organization and the prospective employee. At #25 overall, the top-ranked hospital on the list is Baptist Health South Florida, whose success, they say, "comes from a culture of quality and dedication that is instilled into every member of the Baptist Health family. It is because of their generosity, compassion and commitment to clinical and service excellence that we have a reputation for quality." Similarly, for Southern Ohio Medical Center (#29), "a candidate's fit with our culture is a must! Our recruiters look for a caring heart, positive attitude, dependability, those that adapt well to change, a problem solver, people willing to go above and beyond, critical thinkers, and someone who always tries to better themselves and their team."

The best places to work can afford to be picky, so they highlight the importance of a good fit between company culture and individual employee. But here's the point: If you want to end up on *Fortune*'s list of best workplaces, you can't afford to *not* be picky.

Ten Reasons Why Culture Really Does Eat Strategy for Lunch

Over the course of Sir Arthur Conan Doyle's mysteries, Sherlock Holmes says, "Elementary, my dear Watson!" precisely zero times. Never. Not once. And yet, it is by far his best-known quotation because Holmes himself never said anything that sums up his character so elegantly or so simply. Much the same could be said for Peter Drucker, the father of modern management theory, who is widely credited with coining the phrase "[C]ulture eats strategy for lunch." In fact, Drucker might never have said it in so many words. But the aphorism captures something absolutely essential for organizational leadership today: A focus on strategy by itself does nothing to ensure organizational success. You can have all the cutting-edge business plans and sophisticated procedures you want; if your culture rejects them, they will go nowhere.

That doesn't mean strategy is unimportant. On the contrary, without a sound and coherent set of business strategies, the most culturally vibrant organization in the world would struggle to keep the lights on and pay the mortgage. The point is not that strategy is small or weak, but that culture is immense and powerful. A well-planned, well-timed, well-executed strategy can mean everything to an organization's success—but only if the organization's culture *permits* it. A flawed culture can make a strategy vanish without a trace or, worse, make the organization vanish with it.

Every organization has a culture, but rare is the organization that gives as much time, energy, and attention to nurturing culture as it does to clarifying strategy. You should be as clear, conscientious, and deliberative in crafting your culture as you are in planning your strategies. Be as thoughtful and as careful in designing the Invisible Architecture of your organization as you are in designing the visible architecture of bricks-and-mortar. This effort is the best protection against having another organization's culture "eat your strategy for lunch." The following sections spell out 10 reasons why culture really does trump strategy, illustrated with real-world examples.

Reason #1: People are loyal to culture, not strategies

Southwest Airlines has the highest level of employee loyalty in the airline industry, but its people are not loyal to the company because of such strategies as fuel price hedging, free bags, and first-come, first-served seating. Rather, they are loyal to a culture that honors individuality, fellowship, and having fun. With many experts predicting the likelihood of serious shortages of healthcare professionals in the years to come, hospital leaders should begin working now on fostering a culture of ownership that attracts the best people and earns their loyalty.

Reason #2: Culture provides resilience in tough times

When Starbucks ran into serious financial trouble in 2008, founder Howard Schultz returned to take the helm as CEO. In a remarkable turnaround effort that is still ongoing, the company's leaders implemented numerous new strategies. But what saved the company during its darkest days was not strategic brilliance; rather, it was cultural resilience. As Schultz put it, "The only assets we have as a company [are] our values, our culture and guiding principles, and the reservoir of trust with our people" (2010). Without using the words *Invisible Architecture*, that was exactly what he was referring to. It's clear that the healthcare environment will get a lot more challenging in the years to come; the most successful organizations will couple creative business strategies with resilient ownership cultures that buffer them against the uncertainty and anxiety of a turbulent and hypercompetitive world.

Reason #3: Culture is more efficient than strategy

Another example from Southwest Airlines: During fuel shortages caused by the first Gulf War in 1991, Southwest's employees voluntarily donated money from their paychecks to help the company purchase fuel. The company could have achieved the same end with a strategy of mandatory pay reductions, but that strategy would have come at a much greater cost. Watch the reaction of a typical nurse who has been told to "do more with less" and you'll probably see a gag reflex. At the hyper-successful online retailer Zappos, though, "do more with less" is one of the company's 10 core values. This value has been ingrained into a uniquely positive culture, and Zappos employees take pride in finding ways to honor it.

Reason #4: Culture creates competitive differentiation

At Texas Roadhouse, employees proudly wear T-shirts proclaiming that they "heart" their jobs, and on every shift they stage a pep rally (called the *alley rally*) in the center of the restaurant. Joe once spoke with the senior HR executive at the fast-growing steakhouse chain; the executive said that management recognized that competitors such as Outback and Lone Star also offer great food and great service, but that the key determinant of whether customers return to and recommend a restaurant to others is not food or service quality—it is whether they had fun. And, he said, the best way to ensure that customers have fun is to make sure that employees are having fun. Management has built this culture of fun on the foundation of the company's four core values: passion, partnership, integrity, and (of course) fun.

Reason #5: A great culture can galvanize a counterintuitive business strategy

For every pair of shoes that TOMS Shoes sells, it donates another pair to someone in need. Had either of us, in our graduate classes on business strategy, proposed a business model where one-half of all products were given away, we probably would not have been given a passing grade. Yet TOMS has not only made that model work to create a successful and profitable business, it has expanded the model to include eyeglasses, coffee, baby carriers, and backpacks. If you search online for *careers at TOMS*, the first thing you see is not a listing of available positions—it's a message that says: "Join Our Movement. Build a career that matters and help us improve lives through business." As we've said, great organizations are more than just organizations—at their best, they are also movements.

Reason #6: Culture humanizes strategy

Hospitals across the country are adopting lean process-improvement strategies. This is a good thing, but if there is not simultaneous work on fostering cultural commitment, these strategies are likely to be perceived as simply speeding up the assembly line, creating employee resistance and an increased risk of failure. At Virginia Mason Medical Center, which has pioneered lean processes in healthcare, the lean strategy has been coupled with a no-layoff policy (Kenney, 2010). Healthcare governance authority Jamie Orlikoff is the president of Orlikoff & Associates, Inc., a governance consulting firm, and sits on the medical center's board. He insists that you should not try to fix cultural problems with structural solutions. At Virginia Mason they have coupled the lean strategy with a culture that honors employee job security. Think of it as coupling *lean* management with *lean-on-me* management!

Reason #7: Cultural miscues can be more damaging than strategic miscues

When Dave Carroll, the lead singer of an obscure band from Halifax, Nova Scotia, asked United Airlines to reimburse him for damage done to his Taylor guitar during a flight, he got the runaround. When he threatened to write a song about the airline if his guitar's repairs weren't paid for, he was ignored—to the subsequent regret of management. As of this writing, more than 20 million people have viewed Carroll's video "United Breaks Guitars" and its two sequels, *and* he has written a business book with the same title. Not only that, the Taylor guitar company supplied its own video on how to pack one of its guitars so that United won't break it, which has been viewed nearly a million times! This is a classic case of a self-inflicted public relations disaster. If United had the sort of customer-centric culture for which competitors like Southwest Airlines, WestJet, JetBlue, and Virgin Airlines are known, this multimillion-dollar PR black eye would never have happened.

Reason #8: Strategy can be copied but culture cannot

At one time or another, every major airline has attempted to copy the strategies implemented by Southwest Airlines (some of which Southwest copied from others). These copy-cat efforts have resulted in marginal success at best, largely because they were imposed on a culture that was not receptive. Exhibit A is United Airlines' attempted knockoff, TED. (Remember TED?) Competitors can copy your strategies for promoting a women's health program and can recruit away your best OB nurses, but they cannot copy or steal a culture that wows patients and family members. And if you get that culture right, your best people won't want to leave, anyway.

Reason #9: When strategy and culture collide, culture will win

The preamble to Home Depot's statement of values, which is prominently posted on the corporate website, says: "Our values are the fabric of the company's unique culture and are central to our success. In fact, they are our competitive advantage in the marketplace." When Home Depot hired Robert Nardelli away from GE to become its CEO, he implemented strategies that in the short term increased sales and profits, but at the cost of trashing what had been a vibrant culture of ownership. He replaced knowledgeable long-term employees with part-timers who had minimal relevant experience and centralized decision-making—strategies that violated Home Depot's core values of respect for all people and promoting an entrepreneurial spirit. Home Depot's board eventually realized that by putting profits ahead of people, Nardelli was destroying the culture that had been carefully cultivated by the founders. He was fired (taking with him a huge severance package), and the company has since experienced a strong resurgence.

Reason #10: Culture is an important determinant of long-term profitability

Short-term profitability and productivity are primarily defined by your strategies. Long-term, though, culture has the greater impact. Your organization's bottom line next year will be determined by its business strategies; your organization's bottom line 2 or 3 years down the road will be more substantially determined by its culture. In some of the most definitive research on the subject, Flamholtz & Randle (2011) showed an almost straight-line correlation between divisional adherence to positive cultural norms and profitability within that division. In their study, culture accounted for fully 46% of the best-performing divisions' bottom lines (defined as EBIT—earnings before interest and taxes).

The Perfect Marriage: Culture and Strategy

The ideal situation, of course, is for culture and strategy to work together in a complementary fashion. Grinnell Regional Medical Center, in Grinnell, Iowa, is a "tweener" hospital: too large to be designated as a critical-access hospital that would allow for 101% of cost-based payment under Medicare, but not big enough for added payments that some larger rural hospitals receive. This factor, coupled with unfavorable state reimbursement rates for Medicaid, creates a serious financial shortfall year after year. The hospital has initiated many strategies to deal with this challenge and has received national recognition for being a leader in rural healthcare.

But CEO Todd Linden also realizes that the hospital's difficult financial picture makes it even more important that the organization have a vibrant and resilient culture. As part of that effort, hospital administrators have adopted The Florence Challenge for a Culture of Ownership and have implemented a hospital-wide training program on The Twelve Core Action Values with a group of 21 hospital employees who have become Certified Values Coach Trainers (CVC-T) teaching the course. Todd told us, "The magic happens when an organization unleashes the human potential inside every team member to make a difference in the lives of others. Strong personal values coupled with a sacred mission of service can accomplish wonderful results while overcoming major obstacles."

As another example, Cleveland Clinic has implemented many strategies to become more patient-centered, but none of those strategies would have been effective without a concomitant change in the organization's culture. Here's the back story: Shortly before becoming CEO, Dr. Toby Cosgrove was giving a lecture at Harvard Business School when a student asked whether courses on empathy were taught at Cleveland Clinic. The student said that her father had needed open heart surgery and, after looking at both Cleveland Clinic and Mayo Clinic, had opted for Mayo because the people there had made him feel special as a human being, which had not happened at Cleveland Clinic. Cosgrove realized that his organization "was missing something very important."

Over succeeding years, Cleveland Clinic established the first chief experience officer position at a hospital, had 43,000 employees complete a half-day course on empathy, had physicians complete a course on better communication and empathy skills, and produced two video programs on empathy that have gone viral on the Internet. (By the way, if you can watch the videos on empathy and not be touched emotionally, you probably should work in a field other than healthcare.)

Lessons From the Netflix Culture Code

In 2009, Netflix published its "culture code," a 124-slide presentation that Facebook COO Sheryl Sandberg has called the most important document ever to come out of Silicon Valley (Hass, 2013). This culture code spells out in great detail what the company expects of employees and what employees can expect from the company. It clearly states that Netflix is not for everyone, and that if you do not meet the company's extreme performance expectations, if you are not the best at what you do, or if technology or marketplace changes marginalize your current skill set and you do not grow beyond that, you will receive "a generous severance package" (a phrase that appears multiple times in the document). You might or might not like the cultural expectations at Netflix, but no job applicant should ever be surprised by them.

A number of start-up companies (for example, HubSpot) have created their own versions. SlideShare has created a special page where organizations can post their own culture code slide decks. Clickstop (a company with which Joe is quite familiar) has constructed a culture code to reflect its Invisible Architecture that fits on a single page, as shown in Figure 4.1. (Flip back to Chapter 3 to read about the six foundational core values at Clickstop.)

Our culture of ownership is our competitive advantage.

We must have a competitive advantage to survive.

Competitors can copy our strategy, our products and our pricing. But *our* culture is unique and can't be duplicated.

When we talk culture (how we work), we're talking about our **competitive advantage.**

Leadership is influence.

Some of the most influential leaders in an organization don't have a management title. They are leaders because they see what needs to be done, they're willing to take initiative, and they are able to influence others to work with them. - Joe Tye, Author

"If we aren't thinking big, we are failing our Mission Statement." - Tim Guenther

 Clickstop's Mission Statement: To create a business that is sustainable, enjoyable, and provides opportunity for those who seek it.

Make progress towards your dreams and goals every day.

Pursue perfection, acknowledging that it can't be attained, but that along the way you will achieve excellence. Be courageous and accept that it won't be easy; great achievements never are.

Be your best self – never settle. Prepare for what's next, even if it's not yet on the horizon; your preparation might be the reason it becomes possible. Be strong. Embrace feedback as it will only

make you better. Focus on your strengths, not your weaknesses.

Do the hard things. Speak the truth. Be wise and compassionate. Make time to think beyond limits. Don't make excuses. Encourage others and compliment generously. Be humble. Be honest. Forgive. Learn new skills. Laugh. Have fun. Have a positive outlook. Be grateful.

Courageous
- You respectfully say what you think even if it is controversial.
- You lobby for your ideas, but seek consensus and resolution for the sake of progress.
- You tactfully question actions that are inconsistent with our core values.
- You embrace constructive criticism, and respectfully provide honest feedback to others.
- You take well thought out, educated risks and own their success or failure.
- You contribute effectively outside of your area of expertise.

Strategic
- You seek to understand our strategy, market, customers and suppliers.
- You understand the ripple effect of your decisions/actions on profitability.
- You pursue new ideas and effectively communicate their significance.
- You are aware of how your job performance directly impacts our customers.
- You use hard data and facts to validate theories before making recommendations.

Impactful
- You have a can-do attitude and avoid analysis paralysis.
- You accomplish amazing amounts of important, relevant work on time.
- You consistently perform at high levels so your team can rely on you.
- You focus on great results rather than blindly following systems or processes.
- You responsibly complete tasks on time before handing off to other team members.
- You see what needs to be done and take ownership to make it happen.

Enthusiastic
- You inspire greatness in others with your expectation of excellence.
- You care intensely about Clickstop's success and make time to celebrate wins.
- You have an optimistic, hopeful view of the future.
- You believe in and trust the people you work with.
- You consistently offer encouragement to your teammates.

Decisive
- You can wisely articulate what you are, and are not, trying to do.
- You wisely separate what must be done well now and what can be improved later.
- You make tough decisions without second guessing them.
- You re-imagine situations to discover best solutions to challenges.
- You approach decisions regarding people, tactics and business objectively.

Communicate
- You are a great listener and ask thoughtful questions to help you better understand.
- You seek to understand the perspective or position of peers and managers.
- You are concise and articulate in your communication, written and spoken.
- You treat people with respect at all times even when they disagree with you.
- You remain calm, communicable and approachable in stressful situations.
- You wisely seek other's experience and intellect to find the best solutions to complex problems.

Responsible
- Your coworkers and managers know you to be reliable, honest and trustworthy.
- You have an honest awareness of yourself, your relationships and your performance.
- You are aware of how your attitude and emotions affect those around you.
- You don't offer excuses, and you don't accept them.
- You make time to reflect on your past performance, learning, improving and growing from it.
- You know your strengths, and those of your team, and utilize them in your work.

Opportunistic
- You collaborate and proactively share information.
- You adapt quickly to changes in company structure, market trends, technology, etc.
- You minimize complexity and find ways to simplify processes, keeping us nimble.
- You see challenges as opportunities and prepare for what's next.
- You cultivate relationships with coworkers, management, vendors and customers.
- You recognize when opportunities occur and take ownership on them.

Curious
- You learn rapidly and eagerly, and stay flexible in your approach and findings.
- You question existing methods and recommend better approaches when necessary.
- You look for alternative solutions by asking, Why? What if? How?
- You get beyond treating symptoms and suggesting "band-aid" fixes.
- You look for ways to learn and improve so that you can contribute at a higher level.

Powerfully, genuinely true.

Figure 4.1 *Clickstop designed its culture code to fit on one page.*

Clickstop is consistently ranked as one of Iowa's fastest-growing companies and as one of the "Coolest Places to Work" in eastern Iowa's business corridor. Another Iowa-based corporation that has cracked the culture code is MediRevv, which provides revenue cycle services for hospitals. The company has earned its way onto multiple rosters for being both fastest growing and a best place to work. A blog post describing the reasons for the success of MediRevv states: "The best team members have purpose, and the best leaders provide their teams with a purpose. Following this line, recruiting and promoting based on purpose actually strengthens our brand. This last point falls in step perfectly with our brand concept, that clients choose MediRevv because of what we believe, not what we 'sell'—it's our clear approach, our commitment to results and most importantly, the trust we place in our educated, compassionate employees that set us apart."

Healthcare organizations have much to learn from young start-up companies whose leaders seem to intuitively understand the importance of culture.

Questions to Ask About Your Organization's Culture

- How would your organization's culture be described to a prospective patient, new employee, or physician recruit?

- How can the recruiting and new employee orientation processes be used to hire and onboard people who will fit with, and not detract from, your culture?

- What strategies and tools can be used to reinforce your desired culture, including performance appraisal, budgeting, education and training, formal and informal celebrations, and technology?

- What strategies can be used to engage physicians and other providers in shaping, and taking ownership for, your ideal culture?

- How can you capitalize on your hospital culture to create a competitive advantage in attracting patients and in recruiting and retaining great people?

The 4-P Model for Cultural Blueprinting

Culture is the superstructure of your organization's Invisible Architecture. It's unfortunate that, while almost every organization has a strategic plan, few have a culture plan. But a great culture rarely evolves spontaneously. An organization with both a great culture and effective operating strategies will be most successful, but the healthcare leader who focuses on strategy without also working to create a strong culture does so at the peril of the organization. As David Maister (2008) argues, it is usually easy to see and understand what you ought to be doing, both personally (quit smoking, lose weight, turn off the television) and professionally (be productive, cater to clients, advance your career). Most of the time, you even know how to reach your goals. You don't lack the skills you need to put down a cigarette or pick up the phone, and you most likely have plans to do exactly that. What you may not have is the discipline, the energy, or the motivation to act in your own future interest. Most people find it much easier to avoid hard work now and regret it later.

The same is true at the organizational level. When strategies fail, the problem usually lies not with the strategies, but rather with a culture that fails to inspire people to take ownership for their part in executing those strategies.

The Values Coach model includes four essential elements for creating a cultural blueprint for your organization: Philosophy, Principles, Priorities, and Processes. This structure will help you be more disciplined in your approach to creating a cultural blueprint for your Invisible Architecture.

Philosophy

Start by defining your overall cultural philosophy. In some important respects, a faith-based healthcare system will operate with a different underpinning philosophy than will a secular healthcare system, and a Catholic healthcare system will have a different philosophy than will another faith tradition.

A multifacility healthcare system should have philosophical clarity regarding the balance of centralization versus decentralization. When the pendulum is allowed to swing between those two poles, it is harder for individual managers to know where they stand with regard to decision-making. This also relates to branding. For example, following the merger of Columbia and HCA, there was an aggressive and concerted effort to visibly brand every hospital with the Columbia name. Because of the unfortunate denouement of that merger, HCA has not aggressively pushed for branding of its individual hospitals in the years since. Rather, it has tended to capitalize on the established brand equity of individual local institutions.

For some organizations, commitment to innovation is a key underlying philosophy. Columbus Regional Health in Columbus, Indiana, for example, has established an Innovation Center built around its Intentional Innovation Framework: People, Places, Projects, Processes and Partners.

At any bookstore, you can find both *Putting Patients First*, by Susan Frampton and Patrick Charmel, and *Patients Come Second*, by Paul Spiegelman and Britt Berrett. While the desired outcome of outstanding patient care is the same for both approaches, and many of the practices to achieve those outcomes are similar, the underlying philosophy implied by the respective book titles can lead to very different guiding principles, priorities, and processes.

When Kalispell Regional Healthcare (KRH) underwent the process of redefining its statement of core values, Joe conducted individual and group interviews with several hundred individuals. The statement "Do the right thing" came up in every single interview, clearly indicating that it is a deeply held philosophy at KRH. The organization's new statement of core values concludes with these words: "Above all...do the right thing!"

One of the driving influences in healthcare today is the imperative to move the emphasis from sick care to population health management. Healthcare organizations will benefit from having a clear philosophy about how they approach this sea change in the traditional models. One of the "memories of the future" that Joe created for Midland Health in *Pioneer Spirit, Caring Heart, Healing Mission* is that Midland will be the healthiest community in Texas within 5 years. The health system is now working hard to translate that future "memory" into a reality with a substantial commitment to community health promotion.

Principles

A set of guiding principles puts flesh on the skeleton of your philosophy. For example, a just culture philosophy is guided by the principle that quality defects are caused by defective systems and processes, not by bad people. One guiding principle for an emotionally positive workplace is that jerks are not welcome, no matter how brilliant their technical performance might be.

Priorities

In today's tough and financially constrained healthcare environment, difficult decisions must be made. Having clearly delineated priorities will help to ensure that those decisions are made in the most effective manner possible. For example, in the event of a serious financial shortfall, how will leadership decide among layoffs, across-the-board pay reductions, or other options, all of which are reasonably unpleasant? Or, how does the organization balance the need for high productivity with the fact that patient care quality and patient satisfaction are enhanced by increasing nursing time at the bedside—activities that are notoriously difficult to measure in the quantitative terms of quality surveys and productivity benchmarks?

Processes

A nuclear power plant and an amusement park will share the underlying principle that safety is of the highest priority, but they will have very different processes for fulfilling that duty.

Think about how your organization's philosophy, principles, and priorities are activated through specific processes. For example, at Midland Health, the New Employee Experience includes 2 days devoted to the culture-of-ownership philosophy. Participants receive copies of *The Florence Prescription* (written by Joe Tye and Dick Schwab) and *Pioneer Spirit, Caring Heart, Healing Mission* (written by Joe) about the core values of the organization, and they participate in a class on The Twelve Core Action Values. At Grinnell Regional Medical Center, the performance appraisal process includes assessment of how the employee is living The Twelve Core Action Values at work, and a passing score is mandatory for continued employment (see Figure 4.2).

Section III–Values	Page 6 of 7		
Overall CIA Scoring:	**Green**	**Yellow**	**Red**
■ **GREEN** – 9 - 12 Green and **no** Red ratings □ **YELLOW** – 8 Green and **no** Red ratings ■ **RED** – 7 or less Green and/or **any** Red ratings	★ High Performance	▽ Cautionary	⬣ Unacceptable
I am committed to creating an enhanced healthcare environment by practicing GRMC's core values of authenticity, integrity, awareness, courage, perseverance, faith, purpose, vision, focus, enthusiasm, service, and leadership. I will demonstrate these values in every aspect of my work.			
AUTHENTICITY: Demonstrates self-awareness, practices self-reflection, welcomes external feedback, and positively channels emotions.	☐	☐	☐
INTEGRITY: Prioritizes trust by demonstrating honesty, reliability, humility, and stewardship.	☐	☐	☐
AWARENESS: Practices mindfulness, objectivity, empathy, and reflections.	☐	☐	☐
COURAGE: Demonstrates personal contribution to the greater good by confronting fear and transforming it into determined action.	☐	☐	☐
PERSEVERANCE: Displays a spirit of learning from adversity by preparing for the worst while expecting the best.	☐	☐	☐
FAITH: Builds on inner strength and peace by practicing an attitude of gratitude, forgiveness, and love.	☐	☐	☐
PURPOSE: Lives up to his/her true and full potential while encouraging the best.	☐	☐	☐
VISION: Cultivates creativity, innovation, and action. Displays the ability to recognize a personal role in transforming GRMC from where it is today to the reality of the future.	☐	☐	☐
FOCUS: Is motivated to help identify, concentrate on, and achieve organizational and departmental critical priorities.	☐	☐	☐
ENTHUSIASM: Embraces and encourages a can-do passionate attitude in the workplace.	☐	☐	☐
COMPASSIONATE SERVICE: Recognizes needs and possesses a desire to help and give unconditionally.	☐	☐	☐
LEADERSHIP: Leads by example, exhibits encouragement, sets expectations, and celebrates accomplishments.	☐	☐	☐
Comments:			

Figure 4.2 *At Grinnell Regional Medical Center, employee evaluations include The Twelve Core Action Values.*

The 6-Word Culture Story

In a perhaps apocryphal story, Ernest Hemingway bet a friend that he could write a novel in just six words. He won the bet with this: "For sale, baby shoes, never worn." Hemingway's "novel" has a beginning, a middle, and an end; it leaves the reader with a strong emotional reaction and unanswered questions, which is a pretty good definition of a novel. *Smith Magazine* borrowed the idea and asks readers to tell their life stories in six words (collected in the book *Not Quite What I Was Planning*). One of our favorites, "Cursed with cancer, blessed with friends," was written by 9-year old Hannah Davies (Fershleiser & Smith, 2008, p. 86).

Values Coach has adapted this technique to helping healthcare organizations write their 6-word culture stories. Like a haiku or a sonnet, the story has a precise structure: 6 words, not 5 or 7. The challenge is to actually tell a story that captures the essence of your organization's culture. (This is harder than you might think.) It's easy to rattle off a laundry list of cultural attributes or come up with a snappy advertising jingle, but it's hard to tell a 6-word story.

The paradox is that the stronger and more positive the culture, the easier it is to tell the story in six words. For example, the core values of Southwest Airlines define that company's culture in just six words (hyphenated words can count as either one or two words): "Servant's heart, warrior spirit, fun-loving attitude." Cypress Semiconductor runs counter to the stereotypically laid-back culture of Silicon Valley by calling itself "The Marine Corps of Silicon Valley." The culture of freedom and responsibility that is described in the 124-slide culture code presentation by Netflix can be summed up in these six words: "Netflix employs only fully formed adults." Each of these organizations, using just six words, tells customers what they can expect and tells employees what is expected of them.

Many hospitals struggle with telling their culture stories in just six words. For example, at a leadership retreat at a large academic medical center, Joe broke the audience into small groups and then asked each one to come up with a 6-word culture story to share. The finished products ran the emotional gamut, from euphoria to despair:

We love patients and each other

We are ALWAYS here for you

Multiple priorities, limited resources, great expectations

We're entitled, hating it, and staying

Disjointed departments working against each other

Negativity reigns while circling the drain

I've been here longer; you leave

Beatings will continue until morale improves

The inconsistency of these responses from members of the same management team reflects the fact that the organization had no cultural blueprint, and therefore had not established consistent cultural expectations. And this fragmented batch of incompatible perspectives came from the organization's *leaders*—imagine what first-line employees might have said about their culture. Predictably, the way a person is treated in an organization—as a patient, as a visitor, or as a new employee—will vary dramatically from department to department, from unit to unit, and from shift to shift at this medical center.

Shaping Culture with Bilateral Dialogue

The Women's Hospital, part of the Deaconess Health System based in Evansville, Indiana, has consistently been included in the *Modern Healthcare* roster of best places to work, reaching the #1 spot in 2015. Christina Ryan has been its CEO since 2001, when the hospital was constructed as a joint venture with Deaconess and members of the medical staff. From the beginning, Ryan has been as attentive to culture as she has been to the physical facility. During staff recruitment for the new hospital, current Deaconess employees were required to reapply for their jobs, and interviews for all hires (inside and outside) were focused more on cultural fit than on technical skills.

Ryan's belief that culture is shaped by a two-way dialogue between management and staff is reflected in the way she conducts town hall meetings: "I want people to know why we do the things we do," she says, "so I expect them to understand the bigger picture. I want them to know what's going on with healthcare reform and how that influences the decisions we must make." One way she inspires this dialogue is by quizzing employees on key issues during town hall meetings. When the U.S. economy entered a severe recession after 2008, Ryan conducted what she called "nickel and dime" town hall meetings to discuss the economic picture and solicit cost-saving suggestions. The hospital was able to navigate the downturn without having to resort to employee layoffs.

When the hospital needed to expand only 4 years after it opened, employees began expressing their concern for not diluting the culture by bringing in new people who did not share that culture. In response, Ryan and her team engaged with employees to define what they call their PRIDE behavioral standards, which now account for 60% of employee performance appraisals.

All this work on culture has paid off in a big way. Since The Women's Hospital opened, newborn deliveries have more than doubled, while they have been reduced by more than half at the primary competitor. Registered nurse (RN) turnover has never exceeded 2%, and overall turnover does not exceed 6%, yielding substantial productivity and cost savings for the hospital. The hospital has never had to rely on temporary or agency staffing, and Ryan, believing that her employees are the best advertising the hospital can have, spends little on paid advertising.

In a reflection of the two-way dialogue that Ryan seeks to maintain, she tells her employees to do whatever is necessary to create a memorable experience for patients and their families, and then she asks them, "What do you want to be remembered for?"

Questions to Ask About Your Organization's Expectations

- What are the organization's zero-tolerance behaviors? These should include dishonesty, abusive and bullying behavior, and gossip (talking about patients or coworkers behind their backs), all of which violate fundamental principles of integrity, respect, and dignity.

- What mechanisms can be used to establish these expectations in the minds of employees, volunteers, and physicians, and to teach employees how to deal with transgressions? (In this regard, role-playing is a powerful, but sadly underutilized, training tool.)

- What methods does the administration use to gauge the emotional attitude on each work unit, and what are some strategies to intervene in problem areas?

- How does the organization promote cultural and personal accountability so as to reduce dependence upon hierarchical accountability?

Young People: They're People, Too

You've probably heard silver-haired baby boomers (born 1946-1964) complain about millennials, anyone born after 1980: "They just don't have a work ethic; they aren't loyal to their organizations; they're entitled brats who don't want to pay their dues; and they want to jump to the top of the ladder without climbing rung by rung." Of course, complaining about "kids today" is nothing new—it probably has gone on for as long as there have been kids to complain about. Plato is supposed to have groused, in the fifth century B.C.E., that young people "disrespect their elders, they disobey their parents. They ignore the law. They riot in the streets inflamed with wild notions. Their morals are decaying. What is to become of them?"

Karen Mayer, vice president of patient care services and chief nursing officer at Rush Oak Park Hospital in Oak Park, Illinois, doesn't buy these stereotypes. She finds that while members of the younger generation are more determined to achieve a work-life balance than their parents' generation might have been, they also are willing to work hard and to invest in professional education. They are more accustomed to working in groups and are willing to step into formal and informal leadership roles, without waiting for tenure to accrue. Mayer says that the three key motivators she sees for this age group, the much-maligned millennials, are a sense of purpose and belonging, pride in their work and recognition for their accomplishments, and an atmosphere of trust. At a time when other area hospitals weren't hiring newly graduated nurses, Rush Oak Park hired one-quarter of the graduating class of the Rush University College of Nursing Graduate Entry MSN program, placing many into positions without direct patient-care responsibilities so that they could be effectively mentored on an already well-staffed unit.

> Workplace culture is important to the job satisfaction of all employees. For all generations, the highest indicator of satisfaction is to feel valued on the job.
>
> AARP: "Leading a Multigenerational Workforce" (page 19)

According to the AARP report "Leading a Multigenerational Workforce," Scripps Health in San Diego has become a leader in creating a culture that recognizes the need for different approaches to various generational cohorts. As a result of its work in this area, Scripps has seen increased employee retention, increased numbers of qualified new hires, and higher employee satisfaction scores, as well as reduced turnover and indemnity claims.

Another San Diego company, Karl Strauss Brewing, has a unique approach to attracting and retaining millennials. The company launched a mobile-friendly internal website called House of Strauss that centers around communication, knowledge sharing, and professional development. It also created a rewards and recognition program that promotes peer-to-peer recognition across the entire company and links each individual recognition to one of the company's core values. Team members earn points that can be redeemed in the custom catalog for rewards. The overall purpose is to build pride within the team, create trust and transparency in leadership, and empower team members to be a part of building the company's culture. The impact has been felt across the entire company, with increases in retention, engagement, and a renewed sense of excitement.

Cultural Consistency in a Large, Multifacility System

Ascension is the largest nonprofit healthcare system in the United States. Like other large systems, Ascension has faced the challenge of balancing the unique cultural identities of individual entities that have been brought into the system at different times with having a consistent cultural feel across the entire system. In 2016, Ascension launched a multi-year rebranding campaign to promote the notion of "One

Ascension" and balance the historical brand equity of individual entities and the national reputation of Ascension. The campaign has an external focus on patients and the communities served by Ascension facilities, plus an internal focus on enhancing the cultural experience of being part of the larger Ascension family.

The campaign is communicated internally through a variety of mechanisms, one of which is an *engagement map*, which graphically depicts the complex healthcare environment. One aspect of the map that most impressed us in our research is the way Ascension has complemented the well-known triple aim (launched by the Institute for Health Improvement)—population health, lower healthcare cost, and enhanced patient care experience—by adding a fourth aim, an enhanced experience for the people who provide that care. Nick Ragone (2017), chief marketing and communications officer for Ascension, explains:

> A key to a successful transformation of this size is the ability of a group of broad-based leaders to set aside their individual needs in the interest of the whole organization. The capacity and willingness [of] this group to 'own the whole' rather than their own piece has been a huge factor in Ascension's efforts to date.

The Ascension mission of service to the poor and vulnerable is the underpinning of the organization's desired culture, and caring *for the caregivers themselves* is an essential element of fulfilling that mission. Even in a massive, complex system like Ascension, nothing is more important than seeing every piece of the culture—each individual person, task, and goal—through the lens of overarching order and integrity. *People in unity* is, after all, the simplest definition of community.

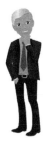

A Note from Joe

I spoke at a nursing leadership event at Vidant Health in Charlotte, North Carolina, shortly after the organization had completed the process of consistently branding its seven hospitals, medical group, and nearly 70 other outpatient and ancillary facilities. Many of those facilities had heretofore been only vaguely associated with Vidant Health in the public eye. One of the comments I heard repeatedly from program participants was how surprised they were by the reach of their organization and how proud they were to be a part of it. ■

The Culture-Building Power of Stories

One of the most powerfully effective ways of transmitting cultural expectations is through the sharing of stories. Some of the world's greatest organizations memorialize, and sometimes mythologize, their early histories by telling and retelling their founding stories. The garage in which Bill Hewlett and Dave Packard founded the company known as HP is now on the National Register of Historic Places, and the company's culture was profoundly shaped by what were fondly known as "Bill and Dave stories." Beauty consultants at Mary Kay are still inspired by stories of their founder, including the one about how she started the company after repeatedly being passed over for promotion by lesser-qualified men in her previous job. In its early days, Mayo Clinic was substantially shaped by the story of how the Mayo brothers founded the hospital after a devastating tornado destroyed much of Rochester, Minnesota, in 1883.

Several of the large Catholic healthcare systems have implemented unique and highly effective mechanisms for sharing stories. Every year, Catholic Health Initiatives (CHI) publishes an ebook of "sacred stories" that have been submitted by employees. As of this writing, 17 volumes have been published and are archived on the CHI website. Dignity Health, through its Project Humankindness, collects and shares stories about the power of kindness. Ascension Health offers employees three stories every day in its online magazine, *Good Day Ascension,* which opens automatically as soon as employees log on to their computers. Twice a year, a magazine is printed and distributed to all 160,000 Ascension employees. These stories do more to describe the employee and patient experience at an Ascension facility than any number of brochures, websites, or billboards ever could.

"We are our stories. We compress years of experience, thought, and emotion into a few compact narratives that we convey to others and tell ourselves...Story represents a pathway to understanding that doesn't run through the left side of the brain."

–Daniel Pink: *A Whole New Mind: Moving from the Information Age to the Conceptual Age* (p. 113)

Linda J. Knodel is senior vice president/CNO of Missouri-based Mercy Health, and is a past president of the American Organization of Nurse Executives. One way she reinforces cultural norms is by asking nurses, "What does it feel like to be a Mercy nurse?" She says that helping them connect their own stories with "One Mercy" nursing standards fosters alignment between the values of the individual and the expectations of the organization.

Although to some people the term *motivational speaker* has a negative connotation, shouldn't that be part of the job description of every leader: to inspire, encourage, and engage the coworkers in their departments? The ability to stand in front of a room and move people—move them to think, to feel, to laugh, and (on occasion) to tears—is a vital leadership skill. Fortunately, it is also a skill that can be taught, practiced, and continuously improved. When managers know the stories and have the confidence and skill to deliver those stories in a compelling manner, they will be more effective in virtually every dimension of their jobs: promoting a positive workplace environment, increasing productivity, recruiting and retaining great staff, and engaging employees in the work itself.

Kennedy Krieger Institute, in Baltimore, which is affiliated with Johns Hopkins University, provides advanced rehabilitation care for children with developmental disabilities. Taking a lead from Story League, a Washington, DC-based company that conducts storytelling events and comedy competitions, the institute has had more than 50 employees learn how to tell a meaningful story in 3 to 5 minutes. People from across the organization listen to coworkers share their stories, often with not a dry eye in sight. One member of the facilities department said, "I always felt like nobody, but now that people have heard my story, I have amazing new friends." Some of the best storytellers at Kennedy Krieger work in environmental services, security, and other departments where one would not typically expect storytelling genius to abound.

The Tornado Effect

In the aftermath of a natural disaster, people come together. Unfortunately, it usually doesn't take long for things to revert to business as usual. We call this "the tornado effect." In the midst of, and the immediate aftermath of, a flood or tornado or another natural disaster, people change. They adopt a spirit of ownership. Nobody thinks twice about doing work that's outside of their normal job descriptions. (No one would say, "Sorry. I don't haul sandbags—that's not my job.") People make "proceed until apprehended" decisions without blaming management or policies for inaction. (No hospital employee would ever say, "I'd love to help you evacuate patients from this wing, but hospital policy dictates that I leave the building if there's a fire alarm.") People concentrate on what needs to be done, without worrying about whether they'll be compensated for it. (You'd never hear an emergency department nurse say, "I know the ED is crunched with all the victims of that factory explosion, but with the hospital's no-overtime policy, I'm afraid I can't stay to help.")

When times are at their worst, people are often at their best. Unfortunately, it's all too easy, and all too human, to forget the we're-all-in-this-together spirit and return to business and politics as usual once the crisis has passed. Finding ways to remember the spirit and memorialize the losses can help ensure that the lessons are sustained, because, as the old saying (often attributed to Winston Churchill) goes, you should never let a good crisis go to waste.

On June 7, 2008, Columbus Regional Hospital (CRH) in Columbus, Indiana, was hit by a flash flood that severely damaged the hospital and required all its patients to be evacuated. The flooding caused over $180 million in damages and destroyed several critical functions, including laboratory, pharmacy, information services, radiology, cancer center, food services, and mechanical and electrical systems. When engineers told CEO Jim Bickel that it would require 12 to 18 months to rebuild the hospital, he sent them back to the drawing board; the responsible teams got the hospital back into operation within 5 months.

In the aftermath of the flood, the CRH culture of ownership was a major factor in the hospital's survival. According to Bickel, the hospital did not lose a single employee it wanted to keep—and was actually able to recruit a team of hospitalists at a time when it did not have a hospital. Hundreds of employees worked in the stifling heat of a temporary tent, clearing mud from pathology slides, cleaning sludge and removing furniture and equipment from the flooded basement, and performing other manual labor far below their pay grades.

The real challenge, Bickel now says, was not in the immediate aftermath of the flood—it was in the year or so *after the hospital's reopening*, when people had to adjust to new facilities, new relationships, and return to business as usual from the adrenalin-drenched rush of recovering from a once-in-a-lifetime natural disaster. During these months, he says, the hospital's values and its commitment to be the best in the country at everything it does were the true north guides that helped it build on that culture of ownership.

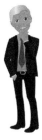

A Note from Joe

As a member of the review team for HealthLeaders Media's then-annual process of selecting America's best hospitals, I performed a site visit at Columbus Regional Hospital and arrived on the fifth anniversary of the flood. I challenged CEO Jim Bickel on the hospital's vision statement stating that the hospital would be the best in the nation at everything it did. He replied that while they would not do everything, for anything they did choose to do, they would strive to be the best. As I made my rounds in the hospital later that day, I asked employees to name whom they personally benchmark their performance against. When I asked someone waxing a floor about her benchmark, she replied, "Ritz-Carlton." In the kitchen, the employee making cookies told me that his goal was to be better than Mrs. Fields. In the years since the flood, CRH has created, in basement space that was once occupied by critical functions such as Lab and IT, an Innovation Center far beyond the scope of what one would expect to see in a rural community hospital—all part of the commitment to be the best at everything they do.

Oh, one more thing: During the year of my site visit, Columbus Regional Hospital was ranked #1 nationally for medium-size hospitals. ■

No Opting Out

If you allow employees to opt out of your cultural expectations—for example, managers looking the other way at toxic negative attitudes because someone is technically proficient in the job—then you will not have a culture of ownership; you will have a culture of optionality. At Midland Health, every staff member is expected to complete the 2-day course on The Twelve Core Action Values; to participate in repeating The Pickle Pledge (see Chapter 7) *and* that day's promise from The Self Empowerment Pledge in daily unit huddles (also covered in Chapter 7); and to think and act like an owner and not a renter occupying a spot on the organization chart.

In 2010, Southern California's Southwest Healthcare System, a two-hospital branch of Universal Health Services, failed a state inspection. The regulators threatened to revoke the system's license to operate, and the Centers for Medicare & Medicaid Services even initiated proceedings to terminate the organization's provider agreement. Morale was low, and the hospitals' reputations in their communities were poor. When new CEO Brad Neet arrived in 2013, he said that "the organization's mission, vision and values were only words on the wall." His team launched multiple culture-enhancing initiatives focused on "building relationships that touch the heart." One of his associate administrators created "I'm In" cards and committed to run, bike, or swim 1 mile for every card that was signed by an employee. A beautiful coffee table book was published, showing pictures of hundreds of employees holding their "I'm In" cards. In 2015 the cultural turnaround was recognized by the Temecula Chamber of Commerce when it awarded Southwest Healthcare System its Platinum Award for Large Business of the Year.

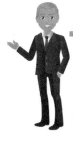

A Note from Bob

Managers can sometimes get caught up in the minutiae of everyday work life and forget the principles of a positive workplace environment. Forgetting their responsibility for promoting a positive culture and employee engagement, they start behaving in ways that reflect toxic emotional negativity. This type of behavior was recently recognized in one of our patient care units. The director and I met with the leadership team of that unit and asked each manager to recommit to the work of creating a culture of ownership. We discussed what this looked like in our everyday work. Every manager was asked to decide whether he or she could make those commitments, and if they could not, were told that other roles could be found for them. One manager who was clearly unwilling to be part of the culture of ownership and refrain from participating in toxic emotional negativity was eventually terminated. ■

Be Inclusive

It's important to reach out to everyone when working on culture change. In most hospitals, the two groups most likely to feel that they are not being included—often, for good reason—are employees who work night shifts and weekends and employees for whom English is not the primary language. In Texas, as in many other states, that can include a large Hispanic population.

Midland Health has made extra efforts to include these two groups. West Texas has a large Hispanic community, and Spanish speakers are disproportionately represented in the hospital's food and nutrition and environmental services departments. With the culture-of-ownership initiative, resources are available to Spanish-speaking employees. Joe's book *The Florence Prescription*, The Pickle Pledge, The

Self Empowerment Pledge, and other key documents and resources have been translated into Spanish. Several bilingual employees have become Certified Values Coach Trainers and now teach the course on The Twelve Core Action Values in Spanish. The Culture Assessment Survey is also administered in Spanish. Interestingly, responses by Spanish-language employees are as positive as, and for many questions *more* positive than, those from their English-speaking coworkers.

Brick Walls and Program-of-the-Month Syndrome

Midway through 2015, patient satisfaction scores began to backslide at Midland Memorial Hospital. The leadership team concluded that, without intervention on their part, the trend would continue in an unfavorable direction. Rather than seek another new "program" for patient satisfaction, a decision was made to redouble efforts on the culture-of-ownership initiative. The Daily Leadership Huddle was established, in which managers recite The Pickle Pledge and that day's promise from The Self Empowerment Pledge; they also made sure that the process was being replicated in unit huddles throughout the organization. The message was that Midland's transition to a culture of ownership was not just a program-of-the-month. It was, and is, a solid organizational commitment reflected in expectations for individual attitudes and behaviors on the job. (If you don't know about The Pickle Pledge and The Self Empowerment Pledge, turn to Chapter 7.)

Shortly after inaugurating daily huddles and other activities to reignite the culture of ownership, patient satisfaction scores began to improve again. There is an important lesson in this example: Whether or not any management initiative, including one related to culture change, has a permanent impact on the organization or is just another program-of-the-month, has far less to do with the program itself than it does with the management team's commitment to the program. Had members of the MMH leadership team thrown up their hands and moved on to another program in the face of 2015's declining patient satisfaction scores, it might have become a self-fulfilling prophecy: "This program didn't work, so I guess we'll need a new one." Of course, no one would have had faith in the new program, either. Worse, the team would have let down all of the people—including the core group of 60 Certified Values Coach Trainers—who have made a strong emotional investment in this work.

Program-of-the-month syndrome is rarely about the program itself. From 2011–2013, the Nebraska Hospital Association and the Nebraska Rural Health Association cosponsored the Values Coach Rural Values Collaborative in that state to make it possible for critical-access hospitals (remote rural facilities of fewer than 25 beds) to share the course on The Twelve Core Action Values with their employees. Three larger medical centers—CHI Health Good Samaritan Hospital in Kearney, Mary Lanning Healthcare in Hastings, and The Nebraska Medical Center in Omaha—provided support and facilities. Over the 2-year period, 20 critical-access hospitals sent more than 150 individuals to become Certified Values Coach Trainers.

As you might expect, there has been a continuum of outcomes. For a number of participating hospitals, the program has resulted in a positive and permanent change in their cultural DNA; others experienced only a short-term impact. The difference was not related to the program, which was the same for everyone, but rather to the commitment of leadership in each respective facility to sustain commitment in the face of other priorities.

The Right Bus Is the Wrong Metaphor for Culture

Jim Collins is the bestselling author of *Built to Last* and *Good to Great*, as well as other books on leadership and culture. One of his best-known metaphors is that the first step toward building and sustaining a great organization is having "the right people on the bus" (2001). This is often modified with the added provision that the right people must be on the right seats on the bus.

There are two problems with this right-people-on-the-bus metaphor, and taking it seriously can lead to serious misunderstandings:

- Unless your name is over the doorway, you most likely cannot choose whom to let on the bus, especially not in the short term. The "right" people might not be available, or you might not be able to afford them. And, in most organizations, you can't just throw the "wrong" people off the bus. Tenure, special skills, HR policies, staffing shortages, and other factors make it difficult (often appropriately so) to discharge employees who seem to not fit on the bus without extended due process.

- "Bus" is a metaphor for a top-down, accountability-driven organization. A bus has only one driver—everyone else is a passive passenger. The driver determines the destination (the vision) and does all the work to get there; the passengers' only function is to sit and wait for the journey to end. It does not matter how engaged or disengaged the passengers are; no effort, or lack of effort, on their part will make the bus go faster or in a different direction.

So, if you can't just choose the "right" people for the bus and throw the "wrong" people off the bus, what can you do? A new metaphor is needed. The best one is the galley ship, where every hand on the oars helps to determine direction and speed.

In a masterful book about the Peloponnesian War, Victor Davis Hanson (2005) describes how the superbly trained, disciplined, and motivated crews of Athenian warships terrified enemy fleets. On an Athenian trireme, every oarsman knew his job and put his back into the work. No one needed a deck master cracking the whip—they were driven by pride, commitment to the mission, and loyalty to their cities and to their comrades-in-arms.

Metaphors are incredibly powerful. The words and mental pictures you choose shape your thinking in subtle but profound ways. Thinking of your organization (or your part of the organization) as a galley ship rather than a bus might open new insights into how the promotion of a stronger culture of ownership can engage every rower to pull on the oars, rather than passively sit in their seats waiting for the bus to deliver them to whatever destination the driver has in mind.

Summary

Culture eats strategy for lunch, but the ideal situation is when culture and strategy work together. A culture code is one way to create a cultural blueprint for your organization. The Values Coach 4-P model uses philosophy, principles, priorities, and processes to help leaders conceptualize the ideal culture for their organization. Stories, including the 6-word culture story, are a powerful culture-shaping technique. Cultures should honor generational differences, be inclusive, and not allow people to opt out.

Chapter Questions

- How would you describe the culture of your organization? What would your 6-word culture story be? Is the "culture quilt" of your organization beautiful and functional, or is it fragmented and dysfunctional?

- How do your organization's advertising, recruiting, new-employee orientation, and other processes work to assure optimal fit between employee personality and organizational culture?

- What strategies and processes does your organization use to make your organization's culture visible and tangible?

- How does your organization engage board members, medical staff, volunteers, and others in the culture? How does it make people from other ethnic cultures feel welcome in your organizational culture?

References

Collins, J. C. (2001). *Good to great: Why some companies make the leap ... and others don't.* New York, NY: HarperBusiness.

Fershleiser, R., & Smith, L. (2008). *Not quite what I was planning: Six-word memoirs by writers famous and obscure.* From *Smith Magazine.* New York, NY: HarperPerennial.

Flamholtz, E., & Randle, Y. (2011). *Corporate culture: The ultimate strategic asset.* Stanford, CA: Stanford Business Books.

Fortune 100 Best Companies to Work For. (2016). *Fortune.* Retrieved from http://fortune.com/best-companies

Gerstner, L. V. (2002). *Who says elephants can't dance?: Inside IBM's historic turnaround.* New York, NY: HarperBusiness.

Hanson, V. D. (2005). *A war like no other: How the Athenians and Spartans fought the Peloponnesian War.* New York, NY: Random House.

Hass, N. (2013, January). And the award for the next HBO goes to ... GQ. Retrieved from http://www.gq.com/story/netflix-founder-reed-hastings-house-of-cards-arrested-development?currentPage=4&printable=true

Kenney, C. (2010). *Transforming health care: Virginia Mason Medical Center's pursuit of the perfect patient experience.* Boca Raton, FL: CRC Press.

Maister, D. H. (2008). *Strategy and the fat smoker: Doing what's obvious but not easy.* Boston, MA: Spangle Press.

Netflix culture. (2009). Retrieved from http://www.slideshare.net/reed2001/culture-1798664

Pronovost, P. J., & Vohr, E. (2010). *Safe patients, smart hospitals: How one doctor's checklist can help us change health care from the inside out.* New York, NY: Hudson Street Press.

Ragone, N. (2017). The journey to becoming One Ascension: Building a unified healthcare brand. In N. J. Hicks & C. M. Nicols (Eds.), *Health industry communication.* Burlington, MA: Jones & Bartlett Learning.

Schultz, H., and Ignatius, A. (2010, August). The HBR interview: We had to own the mistakes. *Harvard Business Review.* Retrieved from https://hbr.org/2010/07/the-hbr-interview-we-had-to-own-the-mistakes

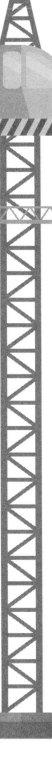

"

We all have the power to decide to live a great life, or even simpler, to have not only a good day but a great day. No matter how long we've walked life's pathway to mediocrity, we can always choose to switch paths. Always. It's never too late. We can find our voice.

"

–Stephen R. Covey, *The 8th Habit: From Effectiveness to Greatness*

The Interior Finish of Workplace Attitude

Chapter Goals

- Explain why culture does not change unless and until people change, and why people will not change unless given new tools and structure and the inspiration to use them.

- Describe the Attitude Bell Curve and the characteristics typical of spark plugs, zombies, and vampires.

- Describe the cost of toxic emotional negativity—to the organization and to the individual employee—and the duty of managers to protect people from its effects.

- Lay out the parameters of the Passion-Performance Matrix.

Core values are the foundation—the heart—of an organization. This foundation gives a solid base to the superstructure of culture. But there's one last element in any beautiful, functional building: interior decor. The interior finish of an organization's Invisible Architecture is *attitude*.

Culture is a product of its people. It is therefore profoundly shaped by individual attitudes and behaviors. For this reason, culture does not change unless and until people change. Have all the pep rallies and programs-of-the-month you want—until attitudes shift and behaviors evolve, you will not fundamentally change the culture.

But of course, change is hard. Think about it: What have you tried (and, to your great regret, failed) to change about yourself or your life? Maybe you've tried to quit smoking, to lose weight, to exercise more; or to stop spending, to save for retirement, to get out of debt; or to network better, to keep up with old friends, to spend more time with family. More often than not, despite your best intentions, you slide back into old routines and patterns of thought.

So, culture won't change unless people change—but people won't change unless they are given some new tools (and, ideally, the tools' instruction manuals). Even more decisively, people won't change until they *make the decision to change*.

You have no doubt heard the saying "Attitude is everything." What you tend to forget is that you can influence your own attitude through conscious choice and effort. It's no easy task, but it can be done. Charles Swindoll's (1990) often-repeated statement, "I am convinced that life is 10 percent what happens to me and 90 percent how I react to it," captures that spirit. While you can't influence world events, natural forces, or even other people's actions on a grand scale, you can dramatically improve your experience by being aware of how you respond to, and gracious in how you cope with, whatever might happen.

In other words: No matter what burdens and constraints the world yokes on you, you always have at least this one choice—a small but invaluable scrap of perfect, unchecked liberty. Famed psychologist and Holocaust survivor Viktor Frankl (1986/1946) put it best: "Everything can be taken from a man but one thing: the last of the human freedoms—to choose one's attitude in any given set of circumstances, to choose one's own way" (p. 86). Many people are far too willing to imagine that there is no choice; that people are who they are, and can't be changed; that you can't choose your own way, but are instead forced down a predetermined path. Others punish people for honest mistakes, and let people off the hook for hostility, apathy, and even disdain.

Spark Plugs, Zombies, Vampires

Data-driven studies of employee engagement consistently find that only about a quarter of employees, on average, are "engaged." Of the slightly more than 100 million people who make up the U.S. workforce, Gallup CEO Jim Clifton (2011) estimates that roughly 30 million are engaged—absorbed in their work and willing to go above and beyond as a matter of course. These are an organization's spark plugs—its go-getters and self-starters. (To some, they are also its "brown-nosers" and "quota-busters.") Engaged employees take pride in their work and draw satisfaction from their jobs; they tend to be more loyal, more productive, and more deeply involved in the organization's mission and culture; they are diligent and scrupulous, but also pleasant and enthusiastic. They don't sit around waiting for someone to tell them what to do—they actively seek opportunities and voluntarily fix problems as they arise. Engaged workers think and act like partners in the enterprise. They are such a valuable commodity, Clifton suggests, that if their population suddenly doubled from 30 to 60 million, the resulting explosion of occupational competence "would change the face of America more than any leadership institution, trillions of stimulus dollars, or any law or policy imaginable" (2011, p. 105).

Another 60% of workers are "not engaged" (or "disengaged"). Think of them as zombies: They punch in at the last second, lurch through the day on autopilot, and punch out the instant their shift ends. Zombies are often competent, but they make little or no contribution to innovation and improvement. The zombie thinks of the job description as a ceiling, not a floor: It defines the basic requirements of the job but also places a hard limit on the work the employee will consent to perform. The disengaged worker is a hired hand, renting a spot on the organizational chart until something better comes along. This person's rallying cry is "Not my job" (or, in the Veterans Health Administration, "Above my pay grade"). In our experience, however, many of these people really want to be (and might already see themselves as) vibrant, superstar employees. One of the most rewarding experiences that leaders can have is to help their employees improve their performances (and their lives) by changing their attitudes.

If that were the end of the story, the sailing would be pretty smooth for most organizations. Unfortunately, the remaining 15% of workers are "actively disengaged." It's an astonishing statistic—around 20 million Americans are "extremely miserable" at their jobs. Actively disengaged workers are neither pleasant nor enthusiastic, neither loyal nor proud, neither absorbed nor productive. They are, in other words, *vampires*: They suck the energy out of the organization, suck the joy out of the work, and suck the life out of the people around them.

The emotional vampire is a leading cause of headaches in managers. Vampires are much more likely than their peers to steal, to slack off, to call in sick, and to quit without warning (or to quit without actually leaving!). Vampires don't cover for colleagues; they point fingers and pass the buck. They expend most of their energy on minimizing the amount of actual work they do; if they are confident no one is watching, they will do nothing—or worse. Vampires' resentment of the job runs so deep that they look for every opportunity to undermine and sabotage the smooth functioning of the organization. Clifton puts it like this: "Whatever the engaged do, the actively disengaged seek to undo, and that includes problem solving, innovation, and creating new customers" (2011, p. 102).

Toxic emotional negativity describes the kinds of ugly, unpleasant, and aggressive attitudes and behaviors often exhibited by miserable people: chronic complaining, gossip and rumormongering, passive-aggressiveness, resistance to change, cynicism, irrational pessimism, incivility, bullying, and lateral violence. In all its forms, toxic emotional negativity exacts an enormous toll on employee morale, patient satisfaction, productivity, and virtually every other operating parameter. It is a leading contributor to stress and burnout, compassion fatigue, and costly, unwanted turnover. Because emotions are contagious, a toxic healthcare workplace can actually cause emotional harm to patients.

Unfortunately, when it comes to dealing with toxic emotional negativity in the workplace, many healthcare leaders droop into a posture of learned helplessness. They sigh wistfully and say, "You can't change human nature." Chronic complainers, cynical naysayers, and even serial bullies are let off the hook because, after all, "That's just the way they are."

But toxic emotional negativity is not a genetic predisposition, or a curse of fate; it is a choice. When leaders and managers look the other way, when they tolerate emotional negativity, when they enable bullies, empower gossips, and tolerate lateral violence in the name of "human nature," they do a disservice to the organization's mission of service and to the profession's ideal of healing. It is a leadership imperative to create a workplace environment in which such practices are not tolerated.

The distribution of engaged spark plugs, unengaged zombies, and disengaged vampires within the organization creates an Attitude Bell Curve, shown in Figure 5.1. The cultural imperative is to shift the shape of your curve from left (disengaged vampires) to right (engaged spark plugs). This requires hierarchical accountability—managers holding employees to appropriate expectations and terminating individuals who refuse to live up to those standards; cultural accountability—employees holding each other accountable for treating people with respect and for bringing positive attitudes to the workplace; and personal accountability—inspiring people to hold themselves accountable for being their best selves at work.

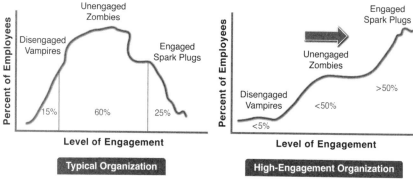

Figure 5.1   *Shift your Attitude Bell Curve from negative to positive.*

The Values Coach Culture Assessment Survey

Values Coach conducts a Culture Assessment Survey, which asks employees of client organizations to share their perceptions of that organization's culture. One of the most important questions asks people to assess, on a 5-point scale, the degree to which their coworkers "reflect positive attitudes, treat others with respect, and refrain from complaining, gossiping, or pointing fingers." As shown in the following chart, when we collated survey responses from 42 hospitals, healthcare systems, and healthcare professional associations taken during 2015 and 2016 with responses from more than 11,000 employees, more people disagreed than agreed with that statement, and less than 5% strongly agreed.

This is one more symptom of "the healthcare crisis within." If, instead of 5%, 95% of respondents strongly agreed with this statement, incivility and bullying would never be seen in healthcare settings. In fact, if that were the case, the words *healthcare crisis* would never be uttered at all.

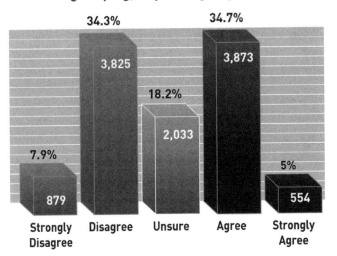

Our people reflect positive attitudes, treat others with respect, and refrain from complaining, gossiping, or pointing fingers.

Strongly Disagree	Disagree	Unsure	Agree	Strongly Agree
7.9%	34.3%	18.2%	34.7%	5%
879	3,825	2,033	3,873	554

Total of 11,164 responses from 43 different hospitals and healthcare professional associations*

* Percentages do not total 100% due to rounding

Values Coach Culture Assessment Surveys at client organizations indicate that the cost of toxic emotional negativity and disengagement ranges from hundreds of thousands of dollars for a small critical-access hospital to tens of millions of dollars for a larger medical center and hundreds of millions of dollars for a large healthcare system. It also suggests that many senior healthcare executives are wearing rose-colored glasses when they speak about how positive their organizational cultures are.

The Hidden Cost of Toxic Emotional Negativity

Employee disengagement costs the American economy somewhere in the neighborhood of $500 billion per year (Clifton, 2011). Because healthcare accounts for nearly 20% of GDP, a straight extrapolation suggests that employee disengagement costs healthcare organizations close to $100 billion per year. A recent study estimates that in the average organization, the cost of emotional toxicity is more than $12,000 per year per employee (Housman & Minor, 2015). But on top of what it costs in dollars, toxic emotional negativity imposes a significant tax on other facets of the organization, as well as on the people who work there.

Emotional vampires often have domineering personalities, which means that they exert disproportionate negative peer pressure in their work units, and disproportionately influence public perception of the organization; typically, for the worse. Actively disengaged workers aren't just a burden on colleagues and a drain on resources (though they are those things). As Clifton points out, "Miserable employees create miserable customers" (2011, p. 99). Customer misery is a particularly acute problem in healthcare because patients are often already stressed, anxious, and/or suffering, even under top-notch care. In fact, vampirism is downright dangerous: Actively disengaged workers are less careful and more prone to accidents and oversights. For these reasons, Clifton writes, "[A] miserable employee, particularly a miserable manager, is a defect—a defect for the company, the customer, and ultimately the country" (2011, p. 100). They are like parasites drawing a paycheck but actually working against the best interests of their host.

A single emotional vampire can have a seriously negative impact on the emotional environment of a workplace: "Avoiding a toxic worker (or converting him to an average worker) enhances performance to a much greater extent than replacing an average worker with a superstar worker" (Housman & Minor, 2015, p. 1). Such toxicity registers in lower patient satisfaction, higher employee disengagement, diminished reputation, greater difficulty recruiting and retaining the best people, and increased risk of serious medical errors. Rudeness, hostility, and aggression can be psychologically destabilizing. They sap your reserves of energy and attention, writes Christine Porath (2015): "[P]eople working in an environment characterized by incivility miss information that is right in front of them. They are no longer able to process it as well or as efficiently as they would otherwise." And this is a disturbingly common phenomenon. According to a survey of more than 4,500 healthcare professionals, "71 percent tied disruptive behavior, such as abusive, condescending or insulting personal conduct, to medical errors, and 27 percent tied such behavior to patient deaths" (Porath, 2015).

Emotional toxicity can easily poison the workplace climate, but it is almost as certain to poison its host. An abundance of research shows a correlation between chronic negativity and job dissatisfaction. Negative thought patterns are self-reinforcing. It is not possible to feel professionally fulfilled and purposeful while at the same time feeling contempt, rage, disgust, hatred, shame, futility, or any other acute and persistent negative emotion. Such workplace dissatisfaction and disengagement, writes psychiatrist Edward Hallowell (2010), is "one of the chief causes of underachievement and depression."

Disengagement is also strongly correlated to dysfunctional relationships outside of the workplace. This makes intuitive sense. The people who are the most negative at work also tend to be the ones in awful relationships, over their heads in debt, or bouncing from one personal crisis to the next. Americans spend more than $10 billion per year on antidepressants. (In fact, antidepressants are the class of medication most commonly prescribed by employee health programs.) There is, of course, no magic bullet or foolproof quick-fix for depression, and medication is invaluable for a great many people. Hallowell's point is not to blame depressed people for their depression, but rather to help them overcome their disconnection.

Bullies: The Wicked Witch of the Workplace

The Wicked Witch of the West is a quintessential prototype of the workplace bully, in several ways:

- Like the Wicked Witch, the workplace bully preys on employees who are new and/or different. ("I'll get you, my pretty" could be their mantra.) This is the reason one hears such things as "Nurses eat their young." It is a manager's paramount responsibility to protect employees—and particularly, inexperienced or vulnerable employees—from such predatory attacks.

- While bullies often seem to be popular, in many cases their apparent hangers-on are actually terrified and praying for someone to intervene for their protection. When a manager finally disciplines the bully, the bully's former followers often say, "It's about time" (and then perhaps launch into a round of "Ding Dong, the Witch Is Dead").

Unfortunately, healthcare's typically hierarchical management structure makes it susceptible to abuse with impunity. According to employee relations expert Dana Wilkie (2016), "Bullying often occurs in workplaces where highly powerful people—or those with high-profile jobs—work alongside those with lower status." Wilkie points to education and healthcare as two fields where this is especially the case.

Cole Edmonson is chief nursing officer at Texas Health Presbyterian Hospital in Dallas, Texas. His successful campaign for a spot on the board of the American Organization of Nurse Executives emphasized the need to end bullying in nursing. Following the election he said, "The call to end this silent epidemic in our profession has been heard loud and clear. It is time we turn our caring behaviors more fully toward our colleagues and those we work with and demand a stop to any form of violence that occurs in any setting." He told us that the Stop Bullying Toolkit has been downloaded over 200,000 times in 58 countries and translated into practice in hundreds of settings across the United States and world. It can be downloaded at www.stopbullyingtoolkit.org.

The prevalence of lateral violence in nursing is reflected in the steady stream of recently published books, articles, and blog posts decrying bullying in the workplace. Indeed, we found 115 articles in the literature with the word *bullying* in the title over the past 5 years—and that was just in the nursing literature.

Literature on Bullying

As important as the books mentioned in this sidebar are, their titles reflect a real and serious problem in the nursing profession in particular and in healthcare organizations in general. Unfortunately, it does not take very many bullies to pollute the culture of an entire work unit; in fact, just one person can do it. The widespread existence of toxicity, hostility, incivility, bullying, lateral violence, and professional sabotage speaks to a national healthcare culture that needs healing.

- *Toxic Nursing: Managing Bullying, Bad Attitudes, and Total Turmoil* (Cheryl Dellasega and Rebecca Volpe)

- *Ending Nurse-to-Nurse Hostility: Why Nurses Eat Their Young and Each Other* (Kathleen Bartholomew)

- *"Do No Harm" Applies to Nurses Too!: Strategies to Protect and Bully-Proof Yourself at Work* (Renee Thompson)

continues

- *When Nurses Hurt Nurses: Recognizing and Overcoming the Cycle of Bullying* (Cheryl Dellasega)
- *Creating and Sustaining Civility in Nursing Education* (Cynthia Clark)
- *Sabotage!: How to Deal with the Pit Bulls, Skunks, Snakes, Scorpions & Slugs in the Health Care Workplace* (Judith Briles)
- *Lions and Tigers and Nurses: A Nursing Novella About Lateral Violence* (Amy Glenn Vega)
- *Bullying: Nurses' Dirty Little Secret* (Emma Majaura)
- *The Real Healthcare Reform: How Embracing Civility Can Beat Back Burnout and Revive Your Healthcare Career* (Linda Leekley and Stacey Turnure)

As of 2012, "Roughly 60 percent of new RNs quit their first job within 6 months of being bullied, and one in three new graduate nurses considers quitting nursing altogether because of abusive or humiliating encounters" (Townsend, 2012). The American Nurses Association (ANA, 2015) has deemed lateral violence an issue of sufficient prominence and urgency to warrant creating a "Position Statement on Incivility, Bullying, and Workplace Violence," which states:

"Incivility can take the form of rude and discourteous actions, of gossiping and spreading rumors, and of refusing to assist a coworker. All of these are an affront to the dignity of the coworker and violate professional standards of respect. Such actions may also include name-calling, using a condescending tone, and expressing public criticism. The negative impact of incivility can be significant and far-reaching and can affect not only the targets themselves, but also bystanders, peers, stakeholders, and organizations. If left unaddressed, it may progress in some cases to threatening situations or violence."

Gossip: The Most Insidious Form of Bullying

Gossip is the spreading of speculative rumors about the personal or private affairs of others, often of an intimate or sensational nature. To tell someone that Joan is having a baby is not gossip; it's a statement of fact. To tell someone that you've heard Joan is pregnant as a result of an affair is gossip—and it is dishonest and disrespectful, and a violation of integrity. To tell a responsible executive that you have reason to believe someone is embezzling money from the company is not gossip; it is fulfilling your duty of stewardship to the company (as long as that executive is the only person you tell). To tell anyone else that you suspect the employee of being a thief is gossip.

> " Let's face it, gossip is one of the world's most destructive habits, and we're exposed to it practically everywhere we go and in much that we see—at work, recreation, sports, home, in magazines, on television. There is absolutely nothing beneficial about gossip—it hurts everyone involved."
>
> –Lori Palatnik and Bob Burg, *Gossip: Ten Pathways to Eliminate It from Your Life and Transform Your Soul* "

Spreading rumors about a coworker is one of the most insidious and malicious forms of bullying because the person being gossiped about is not in a position to rebut the claims or share his or her side of the matter. It always creates the potential for negative judgments and labels to be applied to the individual being gossiped about, and nothing has greater potential to create divisiveness and the silo effect than a culture that tolerates (and by tolerating, encourages) rumor-mongering. Most important, the damage done to someone's reputation by malicious gossip can never be undone.

Gossip is inherently dishonest because even if the gossiper's statements are factually correct, as they spread from person to person they become warped into falsehoods. And people who talk about others behind their backs prove themselves to be unreliable and untrustworthy—if you listen to the gossiper spreading rumors about someone else, how can you trust them not to spread rumors about you?

Gossip also reflects a failure of courage. The gossiper lacks the courage to directly confront the person being gossiped about, to ask whether it's true and seek permission to share the news; the person listening to the gossip lacks the courage to stop the conversation.

Talking about a coworker behind his back, and spreading rumors that inevitably become twisted into falsehoods, can do more to isolate and intimidate an individual than virtually any other behavior. And nothing can do more to foster divisiveness, create silos, harm morale, diminish productivity, and create hostile relationships than a culture of rumormongering.

Venting Can Also Constitute Insidious Bullying

It's often said that venting is a legitimate form of complaining—usually by people who consider it their right to dump their negative thoughts and emotions on innocent bystanders, often without warning them of what's about to happen. Nothing could be further from the truth. One often-cited study found that "venting to reduce anger is like using gasoline to put out a fire—it only feeds the flame" (Bushman, 2002, p. 729). Venting may feel good in the moment, but it is ultimately a counterproductive, and even destructive, habit. And while the venter might feel better after venting, the hapless victim is almost certain to feel worse.

In fact, venting is the perfect metaphor for the act of mindlessly dumping toxic emotional negativity onto another human being. Here are some definitions of the word *venting* from The Free Dictionary:

Forceful expression or release of pent-up thoughts or feelings: "give vent to one's anger"

An opening permitting the escape of fumes, a liquid, a gas, or steam

The small hole at the breech of a gun through which the charge is ignited

The excretory opening of the digestive tract in animals such as birds, reptiles, amphibians, and fish

Venting is gassy discharge, and nobody wants to be around your gassy discharge. "People don't break wind in elevators more than they have to," psychologist Jeffrey Lohr told *Fast Company*, but venting anger is "similar to emotional farting in a closed area. It sounds like a good idea, but it's dead wrong" (Vozza, 2014).

Venting is also bad for the person doing the complaining—it produces the stress hormone cortisol, and can, over time, shrink the hippocampus, one of the most plastic regions of the brain and a key player in anxiety management, memory, and learning. So the more you vent the more you will feel the need to vent. Of course, the people you vent upon typically lack expertise to help you with whatever you are venting about. There are, however, people who do have such expertise: psychiatrists, psychologists, counselors, coaches, and ministers have all been trained to help people cope—and they are the ones to whom venting should be directed, not innocent bystanders in the workplace.

Inspired Managers

It is a management duty to protect employees from the baleful influence of toxically negative coworkers. Someone may go to work wanting to work hard, do a good job, and experience the joy of doing good work in a positive setting. If a manager allows bullies, emotional vampires, and pickle-suckers (see Chapter 4) to deprive the employee of these legitimate rights and opportunities, that manager is failing at an important part of the job.

When a manager looks the other way while a bully abuses a victim, or when a staff person listens to malicious gossip behind the back of a coworker without attempting to stop it, that lack of courage contributes to an unhealthy workplace culture where people's attitudes and behaviors are not compatible with the organization's stated values and cultural expectations. If someone wants to come to work, be enthusiastic and productive, and go home physically tired but emotionally uplifted—but the organization tolerates toxic emotional negativity to deprive that person (and that person's coworkers and customers) of this joy—it reflects a failure of leadership and a sick culture.

The first step to creating a more positive and productive organizational culture is, often, to define and enforce behavioral expectations, including zero tolerance behaviors. A tiny corps of truly toxic people can drag down morale across the board. That is why it is incumbent on healthcare leaders to possess the courage to confront toxic employees, use their management skills to marginalize their negativity, and have the decency to demand appropriate attitudes and behaviors. When the bar is raised, toxic workers either change or leave. And everyone else cheers.

There is good news on at least two fronts: personal and organizational. At the personal level, many of the behaviors of people with toxic emotional negativity (chronic complaining or talking about others behind their backs, for example) are just bad habits, which can be changed. People, by clarifying their own values and dreams, can make impressive attitude changes. At the organization level, when a critical mass of people becomes aware of just how enervating and depressing it is to be subjected to toxic emotional negativity and refuses to stand for it any longer, a profound cultural transformation can occur.

When an organization makes a commitment to promote a culture of ownership, the greatest beneficiaries are often the most negative people (and their families). When a negative, bitter, cynical, sarcastic pickle-sucker manages, through hard work and discipline, to become a positive, cheerful, and optimistic person, the results can be nothing short of miraculous. Indeed, *miracle* is a word people often use to describe the changes that they have made in their lives by making a commitment to live their values.

If we could wave a magic wand over your organization (and your community) and make toxic emotional negativity disappear for 30 days—no whining or complaining, no passive-aggressive victim behavior, no gossiping or rumor-mongering—you would never go back to the old ways (in the same way people will never go back to allowing smoking on airplanes). Why? Because people will quickly appreciate just how caustic those behaviors are when they are not subjected to them day in and day out. They will become increasingly insistent that their leaders provide them with an emotionally positive workplace experience, the way they once demanded a smokefree workplace. The movement will become self-sustaining as you see employee engagement, patient satisfaction, and productivity soar. And as the benefits become clear and more manifest, the movement will become unstoppable.

One of our favorite stories about a leader setting an example for a culture of ownership comes from HonorHealth John C. Lincoln Hospital in Phoenix, Arizona. One day, as the charge nurse group was holding its afternoon staffing huddle, they heard the fire alarm and then an announcement that there was a fire in the endoscopy lab. The charge nurses continued their meeting, assuming that it was either a false alarm or that someone else would take care of it. But then they saw the then-CNO (now CEO), Maggi Griffin, go charging by, in a business suit and heels, carrying a fire extinguisher. She was not going to let there be a fire in her house! (Story submitted by Ginny Schoffelman, RN.)

The Passion-Performance Matrix

The Passion-Performance Matrix is a tool that can be used for both personal and organizational assessment. At the personal level, you are most likely to be your authentic self when you are engaged in work that you are passionate about and that you do well (and are committed to doing even better). You are least likely to be authentic when you are not engaged and not performing. In fact, the amount of time you spend in a quadrant every day is probably about as good a predictor of your success and happiness as you will find.

At the organizational level, the Passion-Performance Matrix is an excellent tool for assessing your Attitude Bell Curve distribution. Organizations dominated by people in Quadrant 4 (high passion, high performance) will always outcompete those where employees are less engaged. This is the secret of superstar companies like WestJet, Zappos, Pixar, Patagonia, and Pike Place Market. The following sections look more closely at each quadrant.

Quadrant 1: High Passion, Low Performance

Quadrant 1 is the "cheerleader" quadrant. Every year, millions of people around the world watch the Super Bowl. Some people are passionate about the game—they wear Cheesehead foam hats and wave "terrible" towels and scream themselves to hoarseness—but nothing is expected of them, they are not accountable for any level of performance, and their passionate cheering has no impact on the final score of the game. Quadrant 1 activities play an important role in social life. Bowling leagues, company picnics, dinner and movie dates, kids' soccer games—these things bring joy and zest to life. But as you know (especially if college was the high point of your life), spending your life in that quadrant doesn't make for a profitable or rewarding experience of life.

Quadrant 2: Low Passion, Low Performance

Quadrant 2 is the "drudge" quadrant, where Dilbert and the denizens of his comic strip live out their lives—doing a lousy job at work they hate with coworkers they despise. They take up a disproportionate amount of management time and energy, and they contribute to poor patient satisfaction, low productivity performance, and low morale.

Quadrant 3: Low Passion, High Performance

Quadrant 3 is the Sarah Rutledge quadrant, named for a character in *The Florence Prescription* (Tye, 2015). Sarah is a technically competent nurse with a negative and cynical attitude about her organization. You probably know someone like Sarah Rutledge, and truth be told, may have qualified for this quadrant yourself at times. Quadrant 3 often represents the greatest opportunity for positive cultural transformation because it does not require new skills and competencies—only new attitudes. Unfortunately, it is often people in this quadrant who behave in ways that are responsible for the metaphor "Nurses eat their young."

Quadrant 4: High Passion, High Performance

Quadrant 4 is the sweet spot. People who do the work to be in this quadrant most often enjoy the experience of optimal achievement, self-actualization, and *flow*. This term was coined by psychologist Mihaly Csikszentmihalyi to refer to the state of total absorption in one's work; he says that it is the highest form of human motivation and satisfaction.

The Leadership Challenge

Your leadership challenge is to:

- Move people from Quadrant 1 (high passion, low performance) into Quadrant 4 (high passion, high performance) through a combination of training, coaching, and setting higher expectations.

- Move people from Quadrant 3 (low passion, high performance) into Quadrant 4 by engaging them in their work and in the organization. If they don't make the shift to this quadrant, they will ultimately and inevitably slip into Quadrant 2 as their negative attitude causes their performance to suffer.

- Give people in Quadrant 2 (low passion, low performance) a chance to improve in both dimensions before giving them the opportunity to go work for somebody else—hopefully, your toughest competitor.

Figure 5.2 shows the leadership challenge in action.

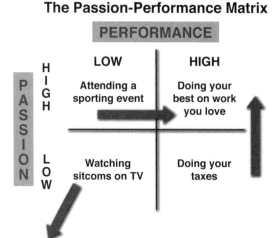

Figure 5.2 *The leadership challenge: filling in the upper-right quadrant.*

Summary

Workplace attitude is the interior finish in the Invisible Architectural construction metaphor. The Attitude Bell Curve charts the prevalence of engaged spark plugs, unengaged zombies, and disengaged vampires in the organization. Toxic emotional negativity is corrosive to the organizational culture. Unfortunately, bullying and metaphors such as "nurses eat their young" are too prevalent in the healthcare setting. Furthermore, venting and gossiping can be insidious forms of bullying. It is a manager's responsibility to promote a positive emotional workplace climate. One tool for doing that is the Passion-Performance Matrix.

Chapter Questions

- Has your organization defined its ZTBs—zero tolerance behaviors—and do managers have the courage to enforce those expectations?
- Where do most of the people in your organization fall on the Passion-Performance Matrix? Where on the matrix do you fall on most days?
- How can you equip and motivate people to constructively confront peers who engage in incivility, bullying, gossip, and chronic complaining?
- Does your organization provide training, coaching, or other resources to help people overcome negative self-talk, poor self-image, low self-esteem, or other underlying causes of toxic emotional negativity and poor physical health?

References

American Nurses Association (ANA). (2015). Position statement on incivility, bullying, and workplace violence. Retrieved from http://www.nursingworld.org/MainMenuCategories/WorkplaceSafety/Healthy-Nurse/bullyingworkplaceviolence/Incivility-Bullying-and-Workplace-Violence.html

Bushman, B. J. (2002, January). Does venting anger feed or extinguish the flame? Catharsis, rumination, distraction, anger, and aggressive responding. *Personality and Social Psychology Bulletin, 28*(6), 724–731.

Covey, S. R. (2005). *The 8th habit: From effectiveness to greatness.* New York, NY: Free Press.

Frankl, V. E. (1986). *Man's search for meaning.* New York, NY: Pocket Books. (Original work published 1946.)

Hallowell, E. (2010, December). Managing yourself: What brain science tells us about how to excel. *Harvard Business Review.* Retrieved from https://hbr.org/2010/12/managing-yourself-what-brain-science-tells-us-about-how-to-excel

Housman, M., & Minor, D. (2015). Toxic workers. Harvard Business School working paper. Retrieved from http://www.hbs.edu/faculty/Publication%20Files/16-057_d45c0b4f-fa19-49de-8f1b-4b12fe054fea.pdf

Palatnik, L., & Burg, B. (2002). *Gossip: Ten pathways to eliminate it from your life and transform your soul.* Deerfield Beach, FL: Simcha Press.

Porath, C. (2015, June). No time to be nice at work. *New York Times.* Retrieved from http://www.nytimes.com/2015/06/21/opinion/sunday/is-your-boss-mean.html

Swindoll, C. R. (1990). *The grace awakening.* Lubbock, TX: Word Publications.

Townsend, T. (2012, January). Break the bullying cycle. *American Nurse Today.* Retrieved from https://www.americannursetoday.com/break-the-bullying-cycle

Vozza, S. (2014, June). Why venting about work frustrations actually makes you angrier. *Fast Company.* Retrieved from https://www.fastcompany.com/3032351/the-future-of-work/why-venting-about-work-actually-makes-you-angrier

Wilkie, D. (2016). Are you in a bully-prone industry. Society for Human Resource Management. Retrieved from https://www.shrm.org/hr-today/news/hr-magazine/0316/pages/are-you-in-a-bully-prone-industry.aspx

Part 3

Values, Culture, and Leadership

"

An organization that develops a strong and adaptive culture will enjoy greater loyalty from customers and employees alike. Cultures that foster ownership create labor and cost advantages because they often become better places to work, so they become well known among prospective employees. Compared with less effective cultures, they generate higher referral rates and more improvement ideas from employees.

"

–James Heskett, W. Earl Sasser, and Joe Wheeler, *The Ownership Quotient*

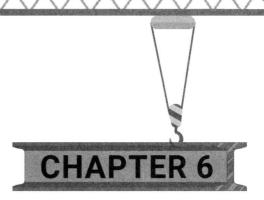

Blueprinting a Culture of Ownership

Chapter Goals

- Explain how a culture of ownership contributes to employee engagement and patient satisfaction, and describe eight essential characteristics of such a culture.

- Share the implicit contract between the organization and employees that should exist in a culture of ownership.

- Show how to utilize the Culture Mapping Schematic Wheel to define specific tactics for promoting a culture of ownership.

I f you could somehow uninstall a healthcare organization's culture, the institutional memory would be wiped clean—a proverbial blank slate. You'd be left with a useless heap of expensive hardware and attractive infrastructure—a hospital-shaped paperweight.

To get rid of a culture, you'd have to get rid of all the people who make it up. People *make up* culture in both senses of the term: They constitute culture, are its component parts; and they invent culture, through improvised storytelling and behavioral adaptation.

Culture is an organization's operating system. Just like an operating system, culture is built from innumerable scraps of coded language that might seem arbitrary and mysterious in isolation. Collectively, though, the culture code serves as a platform for programs and applications. And while some operating systems are elegant, powerful, and user-friendly, others are clunky, wasteful, and unintuitive.

The same concept holds true for cultures. A "shame-and-blame" organization, for instance, will support fear and concealment. The threat of punishment will loom over employees, stifling creativity and discouraging initiative. Managers will tend to interpret this pervasive fear as malaise or incompetence and take an authoritarian approach. The staff will be allowed little autonomy in practice or input in governance. Managers will give commands, and workers will comply.

A culture of ownership, by contrast, seamlessly integrates the three levels of Invisible Architecture. (See Chapter 2 for more information about the three levels of Invisible Architecture.) In a culture of ownership, there is no disconnect between the values posted on the wall and the behaviors exhibited on the floor. There is no conflict or cognitive dissonance, and no coercion or compromise.

Recall the Values > Behaviors > Outcomes continuum from Chapter 3: Core values shape cultural expectations; cultural expectations establish the parameters of behavior and attitude; and behavior and attitude determine outcomes, including employee engagement, safety, productivity, and customer satisfaction. When the process functions smoothly, it creates a kind of upward spiral: Good results hearten individuals and reinforce shared values. Ideally, the process would run like this, onward and upward, forever. But inevitably, some piece of the machinery will wear out or break down, which is why culture must be given constant attention.

Values/Culture Clash

Even the best statement of values is arid and abstract if it isn't directly linked to the culture of an organization and the behavior of its people.

Consider Wells Fargo: Agents of Wells Fargo opened millions of accounts and tens of thousands of credit cards on behalf of customers who had not asked for or consented to them. Authorities slapped the bank with $185 million in fines and civil penalties and ordered its administrators to refund more than $2 million in unauthorized fees charged to customers who were bilked by those phony accounts. Like most scandals in the financial services sector, this Wells Fargo mess is complex to the point of incomprehensibility. It's hard to know who is to blame, and no one is volunteering to take the blame. The bank blames the fired employees; the fired employees blame the bank's unrealistic sales quotas and high-pressure climate (Glazer, 2016; Egan, 2016); and the board blamed the CEO and fired him. As of this writing, Wells Fargo is trying to force the people it cheated into arbitration rather than having their lawsuits heard in the courts; arbitration is far less advantageous for those who have been cheated (Corkery & Cowley 2016).

What is clear is that the company's culture, from the leadership down, cultivated an environment that gave its employees overwhelming incentives to cheat. This kind of behavior should not be possible in a values-driven organization, yet that's precisely what Wells Fargo pretends to be. The company's statement of values begins like this: "Our values should guide every conversation, decision, and interaction. Our values should anchor every product and service we provide and every channel we operate. If we can't link what we do to one of our values, we should ask ourselves why we're doing it. It's that simple" ("Our values," 2016). The ensuing core values, the supposed anchors of all company-related activity, are:

- People as a competitive advantage
- Ethics
- What's right for customers
- Diversity and inclusion
- Leadership

The bank has undeniably used people as a competitive advantage. But has it been ethical? Has it acted in its customers' best interest? Hasn't something gone wrong with the noble ideal of inclusion when more than 5,000 people are forced out? What kind of leadership is this?

The illegal and unethical practices, a former sales rep told CNN, have been "ingrained in the culture for a long time" (Egan, 2016). Still, Wells Fargo's PR machine has insisted on its adherence to its values. After the fines were levied, the bank released a statement that said, in part, "Wells Fargo is committed to putting our customers' interests first 100 percent of the time." Even as the bank was trying to push bilked customers into arbitration, it was running television ads promising to make things right for the people who had been cheated and to re-earn the trust of its customers.

Wells Fargo is an extreme example, and a particular one. Over the years, we have grown less and less surprised by the ethical lapses and valueless practices of financial services firms like Wells Fargo (or Countrywide or Citigroup or Bear Stearns or Lehman Brothers). What does another craven bank scandal have to do with healthcare?

It takes tremendous mental energy and agility to go to work every day at a place that professes one set of values while embodying an entirely different set.

Eight Essential Characteristics of a Culture of Ownership

A culture of ownership is unlikely to evolve spontaneously, but it can be fostered through deliberate management effort. The following eight essential characteristics of a culture of ownership are included in *The Florence Prescription: From Accountability to Ownership* (Tye, 2015):

Commitment: Employees who think like owners are committed to the values, vision, and mission of their organizations, and are committed to their own development in their professional roles. You cannot write this commitment into a job description, but you can inspire it by carrying out cultural norms and expectations.

Engagement: Employees who think like owners are actively engaged in their work and feel a sense of connection with their coworkers and with their organizations. Joe worked with one insurance agency where everyone has the same job description: First and foremost a salesperson, last but not least a janitor, and in between whatever needs to be done. By contrast, Joe once received a call from a distraught hospital foundation director asking how she could prevent nurses at that hospital from removing the foundation's flyers from patient discharge packets because the nurses objected to the mention of estate planning included in these flyers.

Passion: Employees who think like owners believe that their work is important, and they do it with great enthusiasm. Southwest Airlines is an example of a company that has fostered a culture of ownership, with its hiring mantra, "Hire for attitude, train for skill" (hopefully, not for pilots!), and by expecting that people will have fun on the job. In the case of long-term employees who are experiencing burnout, the challenge often lies in re-sparking the initial passion and enthusiasm that attracted them into their professions in the first place.

Initiative: Employees who think like owners anticipate problems and seek opportunities and then have the gumption to take action and seek help if they need it. This is the proceed-until-apprehended principle. At Midland Memorial Hospital, a 2,000-pound happy pickle chainsaw carving greets employees as they come to work. Don Hill, a member of the MMH Respiratory Therapy department, did not ask for permission before he started work on the project; he took the initiative and created a work of art that has made an indelible imprint on the organization.

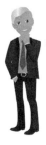

A Note from Joe

My sister Nancy is one of the world's leading authorities on hearing sciences. She's written definitive textbooks, traveled the world as a speaker, and is on the faculty or adjunct faculty at prestigious universities in the United States and New Zealand. But she didn't start that way. Her first job after earning a PhD was at University of Iowa Hospitals and Clinics making $6.50 an hour. Her office was a tiny cubicle across the hall from a janitor's closet. Without asking anyone's permission, she had a sign made that read "Aural Rehabilitation Laboratory" and posted it on the door of the janitor's closet.

When no one took the sign down, she submitted a requisition to have the sink and plumbing removed and the walls painted, and bought some furniture from a mail order catalog. Twelve months later, her lab was on the department chair's "tour" when he was showing visitors around. Nancy's new lab at Washington University in Saint Louis does not need a homemade sign. Because she had a vision of where she wanted to go and was willing to "proceed until apprehended," her lab is now fully staffed, well supported, and provides an invaluable service to the world. ■

Stewardship: In a culture of ownership, employees are as careful with the organization's resources as they are with their own, in part because they know that the organization's leaders are concerned with helping them optimize their own resources. Real stewardship, though, is more than just being judicious with existing resources—it is also thinking creatively about how to create value. Gundersen Health System, headquartered in La Crosse, Wisconsin, has been nationally recognized for its leadership in environmental sustainability. The organization publishes an annual stewardship report, and through its Envision program has turned its commitment to environmental sustainability into a profit center, by sharing its expertise with other organizations.

Belonging: Employees who think like owners are given the inside story regarding operations and finance; hired hands are told only what they need to know to get their own jobs done. Jack Stack and his team at Springfield ReManufacturing (a company that rebuilds diesel truck engines) invented "open book management" to ensure that all line workers understand the company's finances in detail, including how their own work impacts the bottom line—and their paychecks. At Pixar (the company behind *Toy Story* and other animated feature films), the weekly staff meeting covers technology, finance, competition, and other key operating issues; every employee, from CEO to housekeeper, attends the entire meeting.

Fellowship: As we showed in Chapter 5, a leading indicator of employee engagement is whether people have good friends at work. A culture of ownership, where people are truly engaged in the work, is characterized by a spirit of fellowship that encourages friendly collegiality. In *Best Place to Work: The Art and Science of Creating an Extraordinary Workplace*, Ron Friedman describes how innovative companies use physical facility design to create more opportunities for personal interaction. One of the most important benefits of the Daily Leadership Huddle at MMH is the opportunities it creates for fellowship before and after the official gathering.

Pride: Employees who think like owners take pride in their jobs, in their professions, in their organizations, and in themselves. The universal icebreaker question is, "What do you do?" The ideal answer will convey these sentiments: "I love what I do, I'm good at what I do, I'm proud of what I do, and what I do makes a difference."

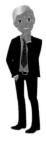

A Note from Joe

I once met privately with a senior executive of a large healthcare system who told me that he never wore his hospital nametag or any apparel with the hospital logo on it while he was out in the community, because he was embarrassed to be associated with his organization. It should come as no surprise that employee responses to the Values Coach Culture Assessment Survey in that organization were among the worst we have ever seen. ■

How does your organization rate on these eight characteristics? Go to www.Culture-IQ.com to complete a short survey that will give you a numerical score and an assessment. If your organization's score is less than 20, you have work to do.

The Implicit Contract of a Culture of Ownership

Based on our experience and research, we have developed a simple implicit contract that prevails in every organization that has a culture of ownership, and that can be used to help guide the efforts of any organization working to foster such a culture.

The organization's leaders promise to:

- Be clear about, and enforce, its core values and cultural norms, and the attitude and behavior expectations thereby established.
- Provide employees with meaningful work and recognize their accomplishments and contributions.
- Help people grow and develop both professionally and personally.
- Provide an emotionally positive workplace where bullying, chronic complaining, gossiping, and other forms of toxic emotional negativity are not tolerated.

The organization's employees promise to:

- Think and act like owners; see the job description as a floor, the platform on which to add their own skills and talents, and not as a ceiling that limits what can be done.
- Take pride in their work, their profession, and their organization, and let that pride shine through both on and off the job.
- Treat others with respect, and refrain from bullying, gossiping, chronically complaining, and engaging in other forms of toxic emotional negativity.
- Be self-empowered and have a proceed-until-apprehended mindset for solving problems and implementing good ideas.

The Culture Mapping Schematic Wheel

The Culture Mapping Schematic Wheel, shown in Figure 6.1, is one of the tools that Values Coach uses to help clients think about what they need in order to promote a strong culture of ownership—which in today's world is the only sustainable source of competitive advantage when it comes to recruiting and retaining great people and earning "raving fans" customer loyalty. You can download this diagram from the resources page of www.TheFlorenceChallenge.com and make copies for everyone who is engaged in the exercise. It is a great way to engage people in this dialogue:

- What are the benefits of having a culture of ownership (the why)?
- What are the specific characteristics that you want to promote in your culture (the what)?
- What actions can you take to foster those characteristics (the how)?

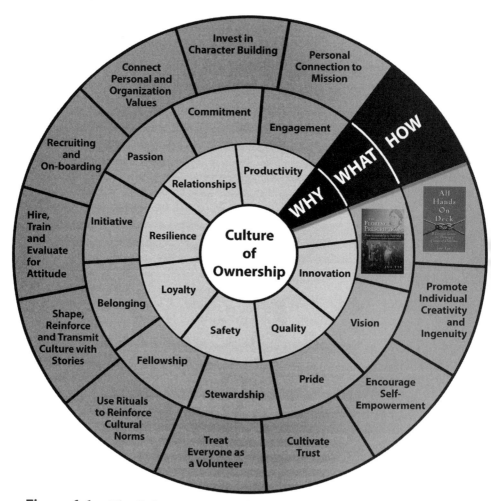

Figure 6.1   *The Culture Mapping Schematic Wheel.*

The Culture Mapping Schematic Wheel is like the lock on a bank vault: You start with the inside circle of the specific outcome you want to achieve by promoting a culture of ownership. Then you line up that outcome with one specific cultural characteristic that will help you achieve it, and from there move on to a particular strategy that will help you build that characteristic. Unlike a bank vault lock, however, there's not just one single combination that opens the door; rather, using a range of combinations will give you multiple options for defining the action steps that will help you achieve the goal.

There are 693 possible pathways through the diagram, and every single one of them can be appropriate—there are no wrong answers. The power of this tool lies in the way it forces a focus that leads to specific and tangible tasks for culture enhancement along the defined pathway.

If small groups in a management meeting or retreat perform this exercise, the distribution of responses can, in and of themselves, be telling. For example, a preponderance of responses that identify "relationships" as the most important item in the inner ring could indicate a strong culture in an organization where people appreciate the importance of maintaining positive relationships. But it could also suggest a weak culture in an organization that does not have positive relationships. One clue to the latter situation is that the modal selection in the outer ring will often be Cultivate Trust, suggesting the lack thereof.

Start with the inner ring, and draw a circle around the salient reason that you need to foster a stronger culture of ownership (in the following example, loyalty). In the second ring, circle a characteristic that must exist for you to achieve that quality of a culture of ownership (in this example, pride). In the outer ring, circle one of the specific actions that can help you cultivate that characteristic (connect personal and organizational values). Then discuss how you would begin implementing that action in your organization.

Inner Ring: Defining Why You Need a Culture of Ownership (Loyalty)

In your small group, lead a discussion on why loyalty is important, including the costs and benefits. If you work for a fast food restaurant with characteristically high turnover, that conversation will be quite different from the one you'll have if you're managing the intensive care services of a hospital, where the loss of a single experienced ICU nurse can result in a five-figure cost for recruiting and training a replacement. For the fast food restaurant, achieving an annual turnover of 25% might be nothing short of miraculous; for the intensive care unit of a large hospital, a 25% turnover rate could be disastrous.

Now consider the factors that are contributing to turnover. Employee engagement and customer satisfaction surveys, results of focus groups, and other data can help you get a handle on what your challenges are, as can comparing your organization with industry benchmarks.

Middle Ring: Identifying Characteristics You Need to Promote to Foster the Culture (Pride)

Having identified loyalty as one of the key qualities you want to enhance in your culture of ownership, look at the second ring shown in Figure 6.1 for the cultural characteristics you need to promote to build that quality. Any one of those characteristics will help you promote loyalty, but for this exercise, select the one that has the greatest potential for leverage. In this example, we selected Pride, which, along with Connection and Trust, is one of the three essential cultural characteristics the Great Place to Work Institute uses to make its annual list. Circle the word *Pride*. Discuss ideas for enhancing pride along these four dimensions:

- Pride in your work
- Pride in your profession

- Pride in your organization
- Pride in yourself

Being as objective as possible, consider the collective pride in your organization along these four dimensions. (Keep in mind that the higher you are on the organization chart, the more likely you are to overestimate how wonderful things are.)

Outer Ring: Selecting a Strategy to Promote a Culture of Ownership (Values Integration)

In the outer ring, circle one strategy you can implement to improve your performance on the characteristic you circled in the second ring. In our example, we highlighted the one about helping employees make the connection between their personal values and the values of the organization, which has been one key to the cultural transformation at Midland Health. Research by Kouzes and Posner (1987) shows that the more clearly employees are able to express their personal values, the more likely they are to embrace the values of the organization.

Defining Specific Tactical Actions (Values Training)

Figure 6.1 has an invisible outer ring. Each pathway leads to a potentially endless range of possible tactical actions for implementation. This step is, of course, where you have to implement a plan. Action is the difference between wishful thinking and positive thinking, between mere good intentions and effective interventions. In the example we have just shared, one way of aligning personal and organizational values (and the way that was selected for Midland Health) is to provide all employees with courses on values-based life and leadership skills. By helping employees clarify, and act upon, their personal values, their values align more intimately with the Midland Health core values.

Engaging the Medical Staff

As important as physicians are to the culture of a healthcare organization, they are often only marginally involved in cultural blueprinting work, sometimes with the implicit assumption that they're too busy or not interested. It is important to find ways to engage providers, and especially medical staff leaders, in questions of culture.

In the implementation of any new IT system, the biggest challenges are often cultural and not technical. A recent RAND Health study found that "for many physicians, the current state of EHR technology appeared to significantly worsen professional satisfaction in multiple ways" (2013, p. xvi). Many physicians feel that a certain electronic health record system is being shoved down their throats, or is forcing them into a clinical decision-making straitjacket. It is challenging to engage physicians in a culture of ownership if they feel that they have lost ownership of such an important element of their practices.

Advocate Health Care is a multihospital, faith-based healthcare system that serves the greater Chicago area. System CEO Jim Skogsbergh made the decision to shift responsibility for both Information Systems and Risk Management to the purview of the system's executive vice president and chief medical officer. While the key motivation for this move was to reinforce the primary purpose of the electronic health record—patient safety and care quality, *not* patient billing—this organizational structure also invites physicians to participate more directly in issues that are cultural at their core, thus fostering a stronger medical staff participation in a culture of ownership.

Engaging the Board

A hospital or health system board should take an active interest in the organization's Invisible Architecture, for these five reasons:

- It will profoundly impact the hospital's competitive position, financial performance, and ability to attract and retain the best employees—all of which are important matters for board oversight.
- In its role as the public face of the hospital, board members should be able to articulate the unique values and culture of their organization.
- Clarity on Invisible Architecture is an essential risk management strategy.
- Culture will have a substantial impact on the organization's ability, or inability, to recruit and retain the best people.
- Perhaps most important from the perspective of a board member, Invisible Architecture determines the sorts of stories they hear from their neighbors at church, at Rotary Club meetings, and in the produce aisle of the grocery store.

The failure to act in accordance with values, along with flawed corporate cultures, can be more detrimental to an organization than flawed business strategies. The board should be engaged in the design of the Invisible Architecture in much the same way that it is engaged in business strategy or the development of new facilities: in an oversight and monitoring role, not by trying to micromanage the operation (Tye & Toomey, 2012).

In his paper "Culture, Good Will, and Valuation," Dr. David Levien, president and CEO of the American College of Healthcare Trustees, noted that a culture of customer service significantly enhances goodwill and valuation; a culture of safety minimizes patient and employee harm; a culture of tolerance facilitates employee creativity; and a culture of diversity helps to prevent groupthink. Members of boards of directors, he says, have a duty to ensure that the executive team promotes these cultural attributes. "By cementing this into the culture, they can not only minimize risk and facilitate compliance but create a true social enterprise" (Levien, 2015).

Engaging the Community

A culture of ownership should not end at the walls of the organization. It's important to seek ways to engage the broader community as well. In Anchorage, Alaska, the Certified Values Coach Trainer group at the Alaska VHA Health System reached out to "adopt" the Anchorage homeless shelter, which was especially appropriate because so many Vietnam veterans ended up homeless. When told that nobody wanted to donate toilet paper because it just wasn't "sexy," the group launched Operation Wipeout; the growing mountain of donated toilet paper in the clinic's main lobby was a testament to employee concern for the homeless of their community and a visible reflection of their commitment to extend the spirit of belonging out to people who had been disenfranchised.

In Toledo, Ohio, the ProMedica health system has reached out to the less-advantaged in that community by launching the ProMedica food pharmacy. By addressing hunger as a health issue, the health system is working to improve the health of its community while removing the stigma of public assistance from beneficiaries. Because the referral is part of the electronic health record, patients who visit the food pharmacy are provided with food options that align with any nutrition-related diagnoses they may have. Patients receive counseling and resources about healthy nutrition, along with several days' worth of healthy food for their households. Patients who are in need of the service can visit the food pharmacy once a month (for 6 months) before requiring a new referral from a physician. Funding support for this program was provided by an employee-giving campaign, one more reflection of the organization's spirit of ownership for the health of the broader community.

Bringing Down the Silo Walls

In the Biblical story, the Israelites knocked down the walls of Jericho with trumpet blasts. At Grinnell Regional Medical Center in Grinnell, Iowa, the Certified Values Coach Trainer group came up with an idea for using shout-outs to bring down the silo walls. With every patient or visitor interaction, employees are encouraged to say something nice about another department. So, for example, someone escorting a patient to Radiology might say, "You are really going to love the way they treat you." This has helped people learn more about departments other than theirs and, of course, the act of complimenting someone else cannot help but influence the person giving the compliment to like the person or department being complimented.

Summary

When there is a gap between the good intentions of an organization's posted values and the reality of that organization's culture, the organization is headed for trouble, as in the case of Wells Fargo. There are eight essential characteristics reflected in a culture of ownership: commitment, engagement, passion, initiative, stewardship, belonging, fellowship, and pride. The Culture Mapping Schematic Wheel is a tool for defining specific actions to promote a culture of ownership. When working on culture, creative ways should be found to engage the medical staff, board of directors, and community at large because they each play an important role in culture shaping.

Chapter Questions

- Complete the short survey at www.Culture-IQ.com; what is the score you gave to your organization's culture? What are the implications of that score?
- Which of the eight characteristics of a culture of ownership does your organization do well on? Which ones need improvement? What steps should be taken to achieve those improvements?
- Which block would you select in each of the three rings of the Culture Mapping Schematic Wheel, and what specific culture-enhancing tactics would that pathway lead you to recommend for your organization?
- What more can be done to engage the board, medical staff, and broader community in your culture of ownership?

References

Corkery, M., & Cowley, S. (2016). Wells Fargo killing sham account suits by using arbitration. *The New York Times*. Retrieved from http://www.nytimes.com/2016/12/06/business/dealbook/wells-fargo-killing-sham-account-suits-by-using-arbitration.html

Egan, M. (2016, September). Workers tell Wells Fargo horror stories. *CNN money*. Retrieved from http://money.cnn.com/2016/09/09/investing/wells-fargo-phony-accounts-culture/index.html

Glazer, E. (2016). How Wells Fargo's high-pressure sales culture spiraled out of control. *The Wall Street Journal*. Retrieved from http://www.wsj.com/articles/how-wells-fargos-high-pressure-sales-culture-spiraled-out-of-control-1474053044

Heskett, J. L., Sasser, E. W., & Wheeler, J. (2008). *The ownership quotient: Putting the service profit chain to work for unbeatable competitive advantage*. Boston, MA: Harvard Business Press.

Kouzes, J. M., & Posner, B. Z. (1987). *The leadership challenge: How to get extraordinary things done in organizations*. San Francisco, CA: Jossey-Bass.

Levien, D. (2015). Culture, good will, and valuation. Retrieved from http://facht.org/aws/FACHT/pt/sp/resources_library

RAND Health. (2013). Factors affecting physician professional satisfaction and their implications for patient care, health systems, and health policy. Research report. Retrieved from http://www.rand.org/content/dam/rand/pubs/research_reports/RR400/RR439/RAND_RR439.pdf

Wells Fargo. (2016). Our values. Retrieved from https://www.wellsfargo.com/about/corporate/vision-and-values/our-values

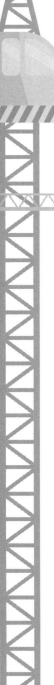

> *Today's best business leaders have come to understand that they can get the best results when they engage their subordinates in the mission, vision, and values of their organization.*

—Paul Spiegelman and Britt Berrett,
Patients Come Second: Leading Change by Changing the Way You Lead

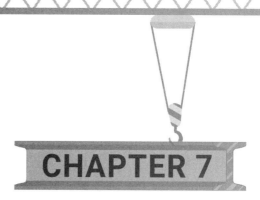

CHAPTER 7

Three Essential Elements of a Culture of Ownership

Chapter Goals

- Describe the three core elements of a culture of ownership: emotionally positive, self-empowered, and fully engaged.
- Explain why toxic emotional negativity—in particular, chronic complaining—is caustic to culture. Describe The Pickle Pledge and The Pickle Challenge for Charity, both tools for promoting a more positive emotional workplace climate.
- Describe the seven promises of The Self Empowerment Pledge for promoting workplace initiative.
- Describe the Midland Health Leadership Pledge as a tool for fostering full engagement through leadership example.

W e have put much thought and study into the question of what constitutes a culture of ownership, including the personal characteristics that contribute to such a culture. In Chapter 4, we shared the concept of creating a 6-word culture story. Our 6-word "story" that describes a culture of ownership is this: Emotionally Positive, Self Empowered, Fully Engaged. We call that The Florence Challenge because those are qualities that Florence Nightingale reflected in her own life and work and that she demanded from those who worked for and around her. At the Resources page of The Florence Challenge website (www. TheFlorenceChallenge.com), you can download a full-color copy of the Certificate of Commitment. Ask everyone in your organization, or your part of the organization, to sign one, and then post them in a place that is visible not only to employees but also to patients and visitors.

THE FLORENCE CHALLENGE
CERTIFICATE OF COMMITMENT

BY TAKING THE FLORENCE CHALLENGE I AM COMMITTING TO MYSELF, MY COWORKERS, AND THE PATIENTS WE SERVE TO BE:

EMOTIONALLY POSITIVE by taking to heart The Pickle Pledge and turning every complaint into either a blessing or a constructive suggestion.

SELF EMPOWERED by taking to heart the 7 promises of The Self-Empowerment Pledge: Responsibility, Accountability, Determination, Contribution, Resilience, Perspective, and Faith.

FULLY ENGAGED by being committed, engaged, and passionate in my work; taking initiative and being an effective steward of resources; fostering a spirit of belonging and fellowship; and taking pride in my work, my profession, my organization, and myself.

Remember that culture does not change unless and until people change, and that people will not change unless they are given new tools and structure and inspired to use them. In this chapter and Chapter 8, we share some of the most important tools that we've used to bring about a cultural transformation at Midland Health and that Values Coach has used with other client organizations around the country (and, increasingly, around the world). As mentioned in Chapter 4, wherever possible, documents have been translated into Spanish for the organization's Hispanic employees.

Essential Element #1: Emotionally Positive

If feelings are contagious (and they are *highly* contagious), joy is "the spreading virus of good feeling" (Goleman, 1995, p. 7). At JPS Health Network, a safety-net hospital in Fort Worth, Texas, CEO Robert Earley has led an impressive turnaround. He has three simple rules that he expects every employee to follow:

- *You own it*. He *expects* his employees to think and act like owners and not like disengaged renters.

- *You must seek joy*. Seeking joy is not optional; it is mandatory. If you can't seek joy in health-care, you probably should be in another field of work. (Note also that he says people must *seek* joy, not necessarily that they will *find* it.)

> " Prying into one another's concerns, acting behind another's back, backbiting, misrepresentation, bad temper, bad thoughts, murmuring, complaining. Do we ever think of how we bear the responsibility for all the harm that we cause in this way?
>
> —Florence Nightingale, in a letter to graduates of the Nightingale School of Nursing "

- *Don't be a jerk.* He expects employees to treat others with respect, to be a team player, and to refrain from engaging in and spreading toxic emotional negativity.

These principles have helped transform JPS from "an overcrowded, poorly maintained facility with an unhappy staff and mistrust among its doctors, nurses, administrators, other hospitals, the hospital district board of managers and county commissioners" into a well-functioning operation that has earned the trust of physicians and employees and the respect of the community (Poirot, 2016).

Derek Feeley and Stephen Swensen, from the Institute for Health Improvement, write: "Caring and healing should be naturally joyful activities. The compassion and dedication of healthcare staff are key assets that, if nurtured and not impeded, can lead to joy as well as to effective and empathetic care… It is everyone's duty to seek out the impediments to joy and then intervene if possible" (2016, p. 70). Again, the key point is that seeking joy is not optional. It is a *duty* to remove impediments to joy, and it is not just a duty of managers—it is *everyone's* duty.

Killjoys

The most significant impediment to joy in the workplace is the prevalence of toxic emotional negativity. By definition, people do not complain about things that make them happy. The more people complain, the more they focus their precious life's energy on things that make them unhappy. Stanford Professor Robert Sutton's research concludes that terminating a toxic superstar liberates the people around that person to such an extent that everyone else's performance increase more than makes up for the loss of the high-achieving jerk. He describes the benefits of an emotionally positive workplace:

Organizations that drive in compassion and drive out fear attract superior talent, have lower turnover costs, share ideas more freely, have less dysfunctional internal competition, and trump the external competition. It turns out that companies can gain a competitive advantage by giving their people personal respect, training them to be effective and humane managers, allowing them time and resources to take care of themselves and their families, using layoffs as a last resort, and making it safe to express concerns, try new things, and talk openly about failures. (Sutton, 2010, p. 170)

Toxic emotional negativity—as reflected in chronic complaining, gossiping, and other such soul-depleting attitudes and behaviors—is the spiritual and emotional equivalent of toxic cigarette smoke in the air. And just as the essential first step to creating a physically healthy workplace environment is eliminating such harmful substances as asbestos and ambient cigarette smoke, so too the first step to an emotionally healthy workplace is raising collective intolerance for emotionally toxic attitudes and behaviors. And, like smoking or working with asbestos, toxic emotional negativity is often more harmful to the perpetrator than it is to the recipient.

Twenty Ways That Complaining Diminishes Your Life

1. Complaining is malignant and contagious and can pollute the emotional climate of an entire workplace.

2. Complaining is depressing.

3. Complaining is an expression of ingratitude.

4. Complaining is an excuse for laziness, avoidance, and procrastination.

5. Complaining is an excuse for the cowardice of inaction when courageous action is needed.

continues

6. Complaining is resistance that prevents you from taking effective action to deal with the problems you are complaining about.

7. Complaining keeps you stuck in the dramas of the past.

8. Complaining is an outward projection of inner negative self-talk.

9. Complaining is an energy suck that enervates you and everyone around you.

10. Complaining is an insidious form of gossip.

11. Complaining is an insidious form of bullying.

12. Complaining is finger-pointing instead of acting responsibly.

13. Complaining makes you boring to others as it causes you to bore even yourself.

14. Complaining is holding on to a grudge.

15. Complaining is parenting malpractice—by your example teaching kids to be whiners instead of achievers.

16. Complaining crowds out compassion.

17. Complaining fosters pessimism.

18. Complaining is the ultimate waste of time.

19. Complaining takes years off your life, both metaphorically because time wasted on complaining isn't really living, and literally because toxic emotional negativity is harmful to your physical as well as emotional health.

20. Complaining is taking up residence in the valley of the shadow of depression instead of walking through it.

Source: *Pickle Pledge: Creating a More Positive Healthcare Culture One Attitude at a Time* (Joe Tye and Bob Dent, 2016).

Attitude

A set of deeply held core values is a (or perhaps *the*) key factor in determining individual behavior, but it is not the *sole* factor. A person who has all the integrity, courage, focus, and enthusiasm in the world but lacks anatomical knowledge and technical skill shouldn't be drawing blood or interpreting sonograms or removing gallbladders. Anybody who's ever given it a second's thought knows that competence has a huge influence on medical outcomes.

> "
> [F]eelings have a say on how the rest of the brain and cognition go about their business. Their influence is immense.
>
> —Antonio R. Damasio, *Descartes' Error: Emotion, Reason, and the Human Brain*
> "

But what about *attitude*? What about the "soft skills" that lie at the very heart of compassionate care? Healthcare takes up the noblest of missions by definition: serving, healing, helping, and caring. Unfortunately, this means being exposed to sickness, pain, and suffering. No occupational field is more stressful or emotionally fraught than healthcare.

A page on the allnurses.com (2014) community forum asks users to cite the skill they found most challenging to learn as students or as new nurses. Some responses mention clinical skills (starting IVs, inserting NG tubes, interpreting EKG strips), but many reflect the fact that mechanical skills were easier to learn than the more abstract duties of patience, conflict resolution, defusing angry and potentially violent patients, fighting for patients' rights, and, perhaps most memorably, the ability to read the minds of MDs.

The list of anxiety-provoking obstacles encountered every day on the floor of any healthcare organization goes on and on: grouchy colleagues, unhappy patients, pushy family members, bossy practitioners, out-of-touch administrators, out-to-lunch managers, limited resources, inadequate support, and on and on. Dealing with people is a huge part of the nurse's expertise—and wherever there are people, emotions aren't far behind.

In the increasingly fast-paced world of modern medicine, time, care, and attention are more valuable and less easy to come by than ever before. Nurses must provide their patients and patients' families with both time and emotional support. Healthcare workers, particularly the ones on the front lines, are often too busy helping others cope to focus enough time, care, and attention on themselves. This is why it is so imperative that every healthcare organization promote the engagement, passion, fellowship, and pride characteristics of a culture of ownership.

No one can accuse nurses of taking the easy way out in their choice of career. According to an American Nurses Association study (2011), 42% of RNs had been physically injured on the job in the last year, and 82% had worked through job-related musculoskeletal pain. A *Nursing Times* survey found that over 60% of respondents had suffered from physical or psychological side effects from stress due to overwork, understaffing, or other occupational pressures in the previous 12 months: "Morale is at an all-time low and I am seriously considering leaving the profession I once loved," one respondent said; "I feel that I am compromising patient care and safety" (Ford, 2014).

Stress in nurses has been shown to have a negative impact on mood and job satisfaction and can lead to depression, relationship disruption, and decreased professional effectiveness. Such consequences are familiar to healthcare workers, not to mention their friends and families. Compassion fatigue. Burnout. Adrenaline dumps. Sleep deprivation. Fear of medical mistakes. Fear of malpractice suits.

But when stress, negativity, and cynicism become default settings—when employees fixate single-mindedly on everything that's wrong and everything they dislike about the place where they work—it is a problem for the whole organization and everyone in it. And it inevitably becomes a problem for employees in their lives outside of the organization when they take that negativity home with them.

Some people will complain to the ends of the earth, no matter how well things are going. It's not a strategy for living, and one you shouldn't live with, in yourself or in your colleagues. The fact is that managing emotions is a skill—or, more precisely, a constellation of "aptitudes for living" (Goleman, 1995). These emotional aptitudes can be improved through focus, diligence, and deliberate practice.

Neuroplasticity: A New Attitude

The new mantra of popular neuroscience writing is synapses that fire together wire together. It means that your brain builds bridges between the synapses that work commonly together so that electrical signals can travel more efficiently between them. The good news is that it is possible to develop new habits—the more time you spend practicing piano or chess or tennis, the more automatic your play becomes—and to break old ones. The bad news is that changing habits is hard work. According to the "plastic paradox," the same neurological properties that enable your brain to change, and to develop new patterns of behavior, can also create rigid routines that are highly resistant to change; because many habits and patterns are deeply ingrained, "we tend to underestimate our own potential for flexibility" (Doidge, 2007, p. 243).

A growing body of research treats willpower as though it were a muscle—easy to exhaust, but possible to strengthen over time. In this "strength model" of decision-making, exercising self-regulation and making difficult choices gradually and temporarily depletes your limited reserves of emotional energy. When your willpower muscle is exhausted, you become less diligent about monitoring your emotions and vetoing the suggestions of your appetites. That's one reason crash diets are counterproductive and ultimately harmful: They often result in short-term weight loss, but the expenditure of energy is unsustainable, and eventually old habits return with a vengeance. Around half of all dieters end up gaining back more weight than they lost (Mann, Tomiyama, Westling, Lew, Samuels, & Chatman, 2007). You may start the day with grand plans for the evening—people to see, errands to run, food to cook, books to read—only to get home after work and collapse on the couch with a microwave dinner in one hand and the remote control in the other.

On the other hand, people who regularly exercise self-control develop more self-control. As with a weightlifter or distance runner, strength and stamina improve with regular exercise. Repeatedly expressing gratitude gradually predisposes you to gratitude (Stillman, 2016). The same is true of compassion (Begley, 2004). Forcing yourself to smile can measurably reduce your physiological stress levels, even if you actually feel unhappy (Kraft & Pressman, 2012). Our favorite example might be that positive self-talk can transform anxiety into excitement: When nervous subjects repeatedly say "I am excited" to themselves before getting on stage to sing karaoke in public, they can actually enjoy themselves (Khazan, 2016). Anxiety and excitement are two sides of the same coin, but where dread is excruciating, open-minded anticipation can be thrilling.

In his indispensable book *The War of Art*, novelist Steven Pressfield calls this "turning pro." He says that simply by showing up every day to do your work, you not only cultivate the inner discipline and personal strength of character that fuels willpower, but in an almost mystical way you unleash unseen forces that work on your behalf (in the case of the writer, he refers to this invisible power as the muse).

Emotional Intelligence Is Resilience

In its simplest expression, *emotional intelligence* is the ability to resist impulses when they run counter to your values and goals. And, as Goleman puts it, "All emotions are, in essence, impulses to act" (1995, p. 6). An emotional impulse can come in all shapes and sizes, from a vague yearning to an irresistible itch. Everyone battles, and in some cases indulges in, his or her own individually tailored set of temptations and vices—sex, drugs, food, jealousy, laziness, or whatever else. Sometimes indulgences are harmless enough, but when the temptation to give in to passions outweighs the pursuit of long-term goals, people tend to act impulsively and against best interests.

Resilience is being tough-minded. Resilient people bounce back from adversity without letting it shatter their self-confidence. When confronted with stressful situations, resilient individuals can lean on coping skills—humor, exploration of alternatives, support systems and relationships, and most importantly, a goal-centered, optimistic approach to problem-solving (Tugade & Fredrickson, 2002).

> Ever tried. Ever failed. No matter. Try again. Fail again. Fail better.
>
> –Samuel Beckett

It's no wonder that pessimists tend to be less-skilled problem solvers; instead of expecting to solve existing problems, they expect a steady stream of new problems. Positivity doesn't just make people feel good; it is also self-reinforcing. Empirical research supports the conclusion that emotionally positive people perform better at work, enjoy more satisfying and stable relationships, and are physically healthier. They are also, it goes without saying, happier (Lyubomirsky, King, & Diener, 2005).

Emotional positivity is the umbrella term for feelings like joy, excitement, curiosity, contentment, and affection. Positive emotions are nice to feel, and people who feel them tend to be nice people to be around. Negative emotions, on the other hand, include anger, disgust, fear, boredom, sadness, shame, and guilt. They are not as nice—but negative emotions are not "negative" in the sense that they are inherently less valuable than positive emotions; on the contrary, both emotional poles are indispensable. Experiencing a negative emotion is a kind of negative judgment, and sometimes negative emotions are healthy and helpful. You don't need to adopt an irrational enthusiasm for the sound of nails on chalkboards, or the taste of rotten meat. Nor should you pretend to be happy when a beloved pet dies. Fear is appropriate when a swarm of hornets is headed your way.

Instead, spend as much time, attention, and effort as possible on cultivating a positive *attitude*. Positive and negative feelings will come and go, but your attitude becomes ingrained in you, as part of your personality. Indeed, it is difficult to tell where attitude ends and character begins. Negative people are defensive, anxious, moody, flighty, selfish, and often just plain *mean*. Positive people are, at least comparatively, confident, sociable, likable, energetic, optimistic, ambitious, flexible, altruistic, and more engaged than their negative counterparts.

The earlier and more often you make the decision to embody positive emotions—to have a positive attitude—the easier it will become as you build up your strength, resolve, and resilience. (The effort to be positive isn't easy or automatic. Sometimes it doesn't work. Sometimes you'll be negative in spite of yourself. But it is crucial that you don't fall into a spiral of self-blame and recrimination. If you fail, and fail honestly, feel satisfied in the experiment and move on to the next challenge. Avoidant behavior always reinforces fear; confronting the object of fear helps desensitize and dispel it. Even extreme aversive patterns like arachnophobia or obsessive-compulsive disorder are best treated through exposure therapy.)

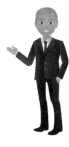

A Note from Bob

At some point, not walking the talk will catch up to you. As MMH has fully committed to a culture of ownership, those leaders and staff who say one thing and then, by their actions, do another, begin to stand out like sore thumbs. At MMH, when managers engage in spreading toxic emotional negativity, they are actively harming the organization—which is unethical; such behaviors must be addressed swiftly. Some people may not know they are engaging in this unethical behavior. Giving them the benefit of the doubt in the beginning and recognizing that people will be, and do, their best with the tools they have, leaders and staff must recognize the behavior and let them know by saying, "That's it! That's what we've been talking about. That is a form of toxic emotional negativity and must be stopped." It takes a relentless collaborative effort to begin eradicating incivility, disrespect, and bullying in workplace environments. ■

The Pickle Pledge (#PicklePledge)

If you walk through the main lobby of Midland Memorial Hospital at 8:16 on any weekday morning, you will see a leadership huddle where, depending on the day, between 50 and 100 people are gathered for a quick update. If you stop to listen, you'll hear the group reciting The Pickle Pledge. If you look closely, you'll see that many (or most) of the people in the huddle are not reading The Pledge—they know it by heart. The way MMH employees have embraced this commitment to transform negative attitudes into positive action has been responsible for significant improvements in both employee and patient satisfaction. It has also achieved something more important: It is helping people be more positive at a personal level.

The Pickle Pledge (shown in Figure 7.1) is a simple (though by no means always easy) promise that you make to yourself and to others—to turn every complaint into either a blessing ("My head is killing me" becomes "Thank God for modern pharmacology") or a constructive suggestion ("The first symptom of dehydration is a headache, so I should drink some water"). By taking to heart the footnote, you also commit to not allow toxically negative coworkers to ruin your day (or to ever do that to anyone else).

Organizations where employees take this pledge to heart are seeing phenomenal culture change. Participating hospitals have seen some of their most negative-minded people leaving—not because of a disciplinary process but because their coworkers simply didn't want to put up with them any more. Employees are making incredible changes in their personal attitudes (and, consequently, in their self-image and self-esteem). Employees have taken The Pickle Pledge home and shared it with family members. One MMH nurse told us that her house was quiet for several weeks, but then, for the first time ever, family members started talking about topics that truly matter instead of whining about the complaint of the day.

I've Taken The Pickle Pledge

"I will turn every complaint into either a blessing or constructive suggestion."

By taking **The Pickle Pledge**, I am promising myself that I will no longer waste my time and energy on blaming, complaining, and gossiping, nor will I commiserate with those who steal my energy with their blaming, complaining, and gossiping.

* So-called because chronic complainers look like they were born with a dill pickle stuck in their mouths.

VALUESCOACH.COM • THEFLORENCECHALLENGE.COM

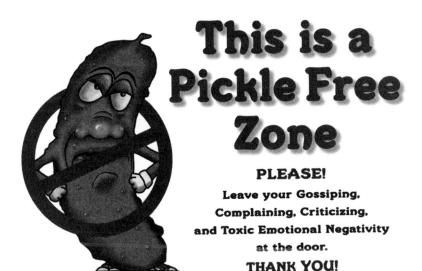

VALUESCOACH.COM • THEFLORENCECHALLENGE.COM

Figure 7.1   *The Pickle Pledge and Pickle Free Zone signs.*

A big part of the magic of The Pickle Pledge is that just by saying the words, you will inevitably change your mindset. If you smile from the outside in for long enough, you will soon find that you're smiling from the inside out!

At MMH, The Pickle Pledge has become a part of the organization's cultural DNA, and it has given employees a new language for constructively confronting negative attitudes and behaviors. Posting signs and door hangers labeled *Pickle-Free Zone* and asking employees to make a donation to the unit's pickle jar whenever they complain gradually fosters a more positive and empowering workplace environment.

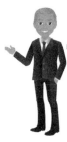

A Note from Bob

At an AONE Board of Director meeting, it was mentioned that organizations that do not allow employees to complain may be at risk with the National Labor Relations Board. The Pickle Pledge DOES NOT mean people should not file complaints about legitimate problems and issues. It DOES mean people with complaints should know how to complain and provide a possible solution in an appropriate forum. Leaders should create a healthy workplace environment with forums such as Interprofessional Shared Governance Councils (organization-wide and department-based) and processes such as Leadership Rounds whereby people can discuss their frustrations and complaints constructively. We spend so much time together at work, we are all in this together to create a more positive workplace environment whereby we can then deliver an excellent experience for our patients and their visitors. ■

The Power of Visual Cues

In their book *Nudge: Improving Decisions About Health, Wealth, and Happiness*, Richard Thaler and Cass Sunstein describe "Texas's imaginative and stunningly successful effort to reduce littering on its highways." The "Don't Mess with Texas" slogan is known by 95% of Texans, they report, and in its first 6 years resulted in a 72% reduction in visible roadside litter. "All this happened not through mandates, threats, or coercion, but through a creative nudge."

This partly explains why The Pickle Pledge and The Pickle Challenge for Charity can have a far bigger influence on actual behaviors than the more traditional approaches of trying to "hold people accountable" for their attitudes. Posting signs declaring one's workplace to be a Pickle-Free

Zone (PFZ), putting quarters in decorated pickle jars as "whine fines," and repeating The Pickle Pledge to turn complaints into blessings and constructive suggestions are similar "creative nudges" that, in a fun and lighthearted way, remind people not to contaminate their culture with toxic attitudes the way "Don't Mess with Texas" signs remind drivers to not contaminate the state's roadways with litter.

An artist's rendering of Penelope Pickle reciting The Pickle Pledge is the first thing patients and visitors see when they go to the Accounts Payable office at Grinnell Regional Medical Center (GRMC) in Grinnell, Iowa. She stands 6 feet tall and is an attention-grabber. She reminds people to be thankful for the fact that GRMC has helped make them better, and possibly saved their lives, and that the people in the AP office will offer constructive suggestions for dealing with their financial obligations. According to CEO Todd Linden, this physical reminder has had a noticeable influence on the moods of people going to AP to pay (or try to get out of paying) their bills.

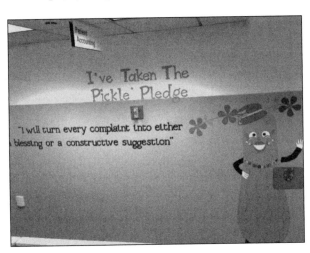

The Pickle Challenge for Charity

The Pickle Challenge for Charity is a lighthearted approach to making people more aware of their own emotional negativity, and that of the people around them, by turning complaints into contributions. The Challenge begins with a Culture Assessment Survey (described in Chapter 5) to gauge the self-perceived nature of the culture within the organization, including the level of emotional negativity. The organization sets a target dollar amount and selects an appropriate charity, often an employee assistance fund or local service organization, to which all funds raised will be donated.

For a period of 4 to 6 weeks before launch of the actual Challenge, employees engage in a variety of incredibly creative projects to promote the activity. At the top of the list is a pickle-jar decorating contest. At Community Hospitals and Wellness Centers in Bryan, Ohio, departments created pickle jars to represent each professional category; several examples are illustrated. Managers and supervisors explain the why and how of the Challenge and do their best to generate positive enthusiasm in advance, in particular emphasizing the personal benefits of creating a more positive workplace by having each individual be a more positive person.

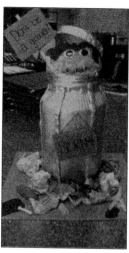 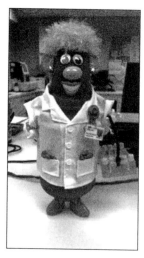

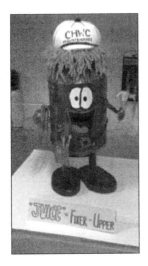
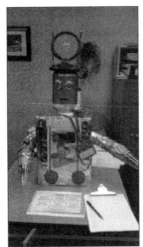

During the Challenge week itself, employees are invited, or volunteer themselves, to deposit a quarter in one of the pickle jars every time they whine or complain. One of the lasting benefits of the Challenge is that it gives employees a new language to confront toxic emotional negativity. We were both in attendance when surveyors from the Det Norske Veritas (DNV) accreditation agency gave their summation report at Midland Memorial Hospital, which happened to coincide with the week of The Pickle Challenge for Charity. All three surveyors commented on how much more positive the MMH culture was than it had been on their previous visit, and they each specifically mentioned the decorated pickle jars they'd seen around the facility. The nurse surveyor said that the highlight of her week had been overhearing a nurse say to a physician, "Doc, you're being a pickle. Put a quarter in the jar." And he did!

The following comment is taken verbatim from an employee evaluation following The Pickle Challenge for Charity at Kalispell Regional Healthcare in Kalispell, Montana. It captures the initially skeptical (and sometimes downright cynical) spirit with which the Challenge is sometimes greeted, the rose-colored glasses with which many employees view their own work units and themselves personally, the gradual unfolding of a new perspective on the emotional needs of others, and the permanence of this new language with which to hold oneself and one's colleagues to a higher standard of behavior.

> "I will admit our unit had a negative attitude about the 'pickle challenge' and pickle suckers. Though we joked a lot about it, made fun of it a fair amount, and balked at the possibility that we could possibly need a change here in our 'wonderful department,' I do see people care about each other a little more, provide patients with a deeper level of care without the superficial caring attitude, and staff take care of the real needs among us that make a difference in the place we work. We are still quick to tell people, 'That will cost you a quarter,' but the understood meaning behind it does change the direction of the conversation, the mood, and ultimately the patient care environment."

One of the decorated pickle jars at Piedmont Fayette Hospital in Fayetteville, Georgia, had a sign that read, "Be brave enough to start a conversation that matters." Complaining is faux conversation, which is often a way to avoid having conversations that really matter because the courage is lacking. It takes courage to deal with problems instead of just whining about them.

The first 31 healthcare organizations that took The Pickle Challenge for Charity raised more than $40,000 for charitable donations during their 1-week Challenge periods ($58,000 including matching contributions from Values Coach). Think of that! In just those 31 organizations, in just their 1-week challenge periods, more than 160,000 times, employees caught themselves or coworkers whining and complaining and put a quarter in a decorated pickle jar. Extrapolating those results to the entire healthcare industry for a 1-year period suggests that if every complaint were turned into a 25-cent contribution, billions of dollars could be raised for charitable causes, toxic emotional negativity could be eradicated from the workplace, and more positive and productive cultures of ownership could be built.

The Pickle Challenge and Hospital Values

The following excerpt from *Pioneer Spirit, Caring Heart, Healing Mission*—the book that Joe wrote to communicate the core values of Midland Health—explains how The Pickle Challenge reinforces those values:

"The Pickle Challenge is one of the most important ways that we live our values…At Midland Health, our first core value is Pioneer Spirit. True pioneers don't complain about things—they do something about them. Our second core value is Caring Heart. How can you create a caring environment if you're surrounded with toxic emotional negativity? And our third core value is Healing Mission…Part of our commitment to a healing mission is making sure that our people work in, and our patients are cared for in, a healing environment. That begins with declaring this hospital to be a Pickle-Free Zone. And it continues with helping the people we serve to have the courage and strength to take care of their emotional health as well as their physical health."

Source: *Pioneer Spirit, Caring Heart, Healing Mission: Midland Health—Honoring the Past, Creating the Future* (Tye, 2015).

Anticipate (and Prepare for) Resistance

You will almost certainly get resistance to The Pickle Challenge for Charity, and it will be most vociferous from people who are the biggest part of the problem. In many cases, it will also be the people who could most benefit personally from having a more positive attitude—not to mention their families at home who receive the tail end of toxic emotional negativity when Mom or Dad comes home at the end of a workday. Stick with it. In many cases some of the people who are initially the most negative will end up being your most positive spark plugs as they experience the personal, professional, and family benefits of taking The Pickle Pledge to heart.

Essential Element #2: Self Empowered

One of the most misused buzzwords in management is *empowerment*. If someone else can give you power, they can also take it away—and loaned empowerment is not real power. In truth, no one can empower you but you. The only genuine empowerment is self-empowerment. Empowerment is a state of mind—not part of a job description, a set of delegated tasks, or the latest management program brought in by the boss. Once you have given yourself that inner power, no one can take it away from you.

To be empowered is to replace a sense of entitlement with a spirit of aspiration, to replace excuse-making with action-taking. It is to empower yourself rather than waiting for someone else to do it for you.

The Self Empowerment Pledge

A spirit of self-empowerment is the catalyst for a "proceed-until-apprehended" commitment to initiative. The Self Empowerment Pledge is a powerful tool for giving oneself the power of self-empowerment. It features one promise for each day of the week (Responsibility,

No empowerment is so effective as self-empowerment...In this world, the optimists have it, not because they are always right, but because they are always positive. Even when wrong, they are positive, and that is the way of achievement, correction, improvement, and success. Educated, eyes-open optimism pays; pessimism can only offer the empty consolation of being right [because it creates a self-fulfilling prophecy of failure]."

–David Landes, "Culture Makes Almost All the Difference"

99

Accountability, Determination, Contribution, Resilience, Perspective, and Faith). Participants are invited to repeat each day's promise four times a day (morning, noon, afternoon, and evening), out loud whenever possible, and in a group setting at least once.

> "
> I attribute my success to the fact that I never gave or took an excuse.
>
> –Florence Nightingale
> "

Here's how it works: You keep promising yourself that you will be responsible for your life, accountable to yourself, determined to achieve your goals, committed to making a contribution, resilient in the face of adversity, possessing a positive perspective on your challenges, and letting your faith and gratitude shine through in your attitudes and in your actions. You're committing to yourself to curb whining and complaining, procrastinating, gossiping, blaming others for your problems, taking when you should be giving, and pretending that you have no power. Of course, if you are paying attention, you will catch yourself breaking these promises with some frequency. The longer you do this, the more likely it is that you will develop what psychologists call *cognitive dissonance*—trying to hold two incompatible beliefs at the same time. This is a form of mental illness!

At that point, one of three things must happen. First, you could decide that you are okay with having a bit of mental illness—you keep making the promises, keep breaking them, and live with cognitive dissonance. Second, you take the easy way and stop making the promises—not because you don't have enough time but because the longer you make the promises, the more painful it becomes to catch yourself breaking them.

Ideally, though, as you keep making the promises and work through the mental pain of catching yourself breaking them, you begin to change your attitudes and behaviors to become more consistent with the promises that you are making to yourself (thereby alleviating cognitive dissonance). As you do that, you will start to do a better job of meeting deadlines, work on building more trusting relationships, fill out applications for graduate school, or whatever up until now you've been pretending that you're not empowered to do. But these promises aren't just for work; they can also help you make a personal commitment to exercise more and eat a healthier diet, be more responsible with your finances, watch less television and spend more time with family, or any other personal priorities. As you start to achieve those results, the promises become part of your personal character DNA because you have proven to yourself that they work.

According to Jeffrey M. Schwartz and Sharon Begley, "[W]e are seeing evidence of the brain's ability to remake itself throughout adult life, not only in response to outside stimuli, but even in response to directed mental effort. We are seeing, in short, the brain's potential to correct its own flaws and enhance its own capabilities" (2002, p. 223). When people consistently say the words included in these seven life-changing promises, they will actually begin to hardwire those commitments into the neural networks of their brains. Words shape thoughts, thoughts catalyze beliefs, beliefs inspire actions, actions build habits, and habits create results.

The Seven Daily Promises

The Self Empowerment Pledge includes seven simple promises that will change your life, if you are willing to invest 1 minute a day for a year. Read these seven promises, and then ask yourself these two questions:

- *Question #1:* If I were to take these promises to heart and act on them, would I be better off in every way—personally, professionally, financially, and spiritually—in 1 year than where my current life trajectory is taking me?

- *Question #2:* If everyone where I work were to take these promises to heart and act on them, would we do a better job of serving our patients and supporting each other, and would this be a better place to work?

If you're being honest, the answer will be absolutely yes—how could it be anything else? The promises themselves are simple, but keeping them will require desire and determination. Fortunately, you don't have to tackle them all at once. Focus on one promise each day so that you make all seven promises to yourself each week. Do this each day for 1 year—it will be the best daily 1 minute you ever invest in yourself. In the following sections, we describe each of these seven life-changing promises.

Monday's Promise: Responsibility

I will take complete responsibility for my health, my happiness, my success, and my life, and will not blame others for my problems or predicaments.

Monday's Promise says that you will take complete responsibility for your life and refrain from blaming other people for your circumstances. Legendary basketball coach John Wooden told his players that no one is a loser until he blames someone else for the loss. Life-altering success only begins when you take complete and absolute responsibility for your circumstances and your outcomes. When you stop playing the "blame-and-complain game" and take responsibility for your life, you're on the road to achieving your goals. By the way, this is an important distinction: a problem has a solution, and a predicament does not. Monday's Promise says that you will deal with problems and live with predicaments, but not complain about either.

Tuesday's Promise: Accountability

I will not allow low self-esteem, self-limiting beliefs, or the negativity of others to prevent me from achieving my authentic goals and from becoming the person I am meant to be.

On Tuesday, you promise to hold yourself accountable—not just for meeting your obligations but also for fulfilling your true potential. In *The War of Art*, Steven Pressfield describes Resistance (he capitalizes the word to denote that it is a real and visceral presence, like cancer or a great white shark) as the inner accumulation of fears and doubts that blocks you from expressing your creativity. "The more important a call or action is to our soul's evolution," he says, "the more Resistance we will feel toward pursuing it" (Pressfield, 2012, p. 12). The key to conquering Resistance is internalizing and operationalizing Tuesday's Promise. Pressfield says that beating Resistance is a fight to the death. Every time you let it beat you, a little part of your soul dies; every time you beat it, you grow a little stronger.

Wednesday's Promise: Determination

I will do the things I'm afraid to do, but which I know should be done. Sometimes this will mean asking for help to do that which I cannot do by myself.

On Wednesday, you promise to bravely confront your fears. Every great accomplishment was once the "impossible" dream of a dreamer who simply refused to quit when the going got tough. For the person starting a new business, it takes time to get the product and the marketing right, to get word-of-mouth working, and to find the right people for the team. There will be frustration and failure along the way—it's all part of the game. The difference between winners and losers is that winners are determined to do what it takes to stay in the game, no matter what the score is at halftime. And they know that to stay in the game, they must be willing to ask for the help they need, because no one can achieve big goals alone.

Thursday's Promise: Contribution

I will earn the help I need in advance by helping other people now, and repay the help I receive by serving others later.

With Thursday's Promise, you commit yourself to paying forward as well as to paying back. As you internalize Thursday's Promise, you will begin to appreciate the ancient wisdom of the Chinese philosopher Chuang Tzu, who said that you can never become happy and successful by trying to achieve happiness and success, but only by helping others to be happier and more successful. One of the great paradoxes of life is that the more you devote yourself to service to others, the richer and more rewarding (and eventually rewarded) your life will be. If you read the book or saw the movie *Pay It Forward*, you'll recognize that philosophy in this promise.

Friday's Promise: Resilience

I will face rejection and failure with courage, awareness, and perseverance, making these experiences the platform for future acceptance and success.

You often hear figures quoted about business failure—for example, nine of every ten new businesses fail within the first 5 years, or something like that. Not only is that misleading (excluding people who are just sticking a toe in the water, the 5-year survival rate for new businesses is much greater than that), it is simply not true. Businesses do not fail—owners quit. For every business that has "failed," there is another where, in the very same dire straits, the owner(s) put in one more late night, made one more sales call, or did whatever else it took to survive that dark night of the business soul and went on to build a successful enterprise. Internalizing Friday's Promise will help you bounce back every time you fall and blast your way through every brick wall.

Saturday's Promise: Perspective

Though I might not understand why adversity happens, by my conscious choice I will find strength, compassion, and grace through my trials.

On Saturday, you make the "silver lining" promise of seeing the best in every situation. One of Joe's favorite sayings is, "Thank God Ahead of Time" (the title of a book by Father Michael Crosby). Bad things do happen to good people: When they happen to you, you can play the victim, or you can say "thank you" and plumb the experience for its lessons. Almost everyone who has ever lost a job will eventually say that it was the best thing that could have happened (the exception: people who choose to play the lifelong victim role); the sooner you internalize Saturday's Promise, the more quickly you will find the silver lining in every dark cloud. If you spend time with support groups, you will be impressed with how people choose to find hidden blessings in apparent tragedy. If they can find blessings in cancer, addiction, or even the loss of a child, what can happen to you that you can't immediately say, "Thank you—I don't know why yet, but I'll figure it out."

Sunday's Promise: Faith

My faith and my gratitude for all that I have been blessed with will shine through in my attitudes and in my actions.

On Sunday, you promise yourself to be faithful. This isn't a promise about religion—everyone, regardless of his or her religious belief or nonbelief, needs faith: faith in yourself, faith in other people, faith in the future, and hopefully faith in things unseen. On the wall of Joe's home office is a shadow box that houses a delicate, handmade paper angel. A dear friend gave it to him several days before she died of cancer, much too young. During her last year on earth, her faith and her gratitude for the blessings of her life radiated outward like sunshine pouring through a stained glass window. She was a constant inspiration to her family, members of support groups she stayed with to the end, and many others, including Joe. Ending your week with Sunday's Promise will remind you to be thankful for all that you have been blessed with. And if you live in the America of today, you have many blessings indeed.

The Power of Groups and Rituals

The Daily Leadership Huddle at Midland Memorial Hospital starts each morning in the main lobby with a recitation of The Pickle Pledge and that day's promise from The Self Empowerment Pledge. The process is then replicated in unit huddles throughout the organization. This group ritual has been a big part of instilling the culture of ownership philosophy into the cultural DNA of Midland Health, and communicating to everyone who passes by that the leadership team takes this very seriously.

This group reading has a double benefit:

- People are more likely to stick to the promises they have made if they've been made publicly (and if coworkers gently remind them of the promises when they break them).

- When a critical mass of people within an organization internalize and act upon the promises, they inevitably have a positive impact on culture.

> There's something really powerful about groups and shared experiences. People might be skeptical about their ability to change if they're by themselves, but a group will convince them to suspend their disbelief. A community creates belief.
>
> —Lee Ann Kaskutas, senior scientist at the Alcohol Research Group, as reported by Charles Duhigg in *The Power of Habit*

Shortly after inauguration of the daily huddles and other activities to re-spark the culture of ownership work at MMH, patient satisfaction scores began to increase again and in many areas are at record high levels.

Essential Element #3: Fully Engaged

Abraham Maslow crowned his famous hierarchy of needs with self-actualization, "the desire to become more and more what one is, to become everything that one is capable of becoming" (1954, p. 46). Even if the other cravings—for sustenance, for safety, for love and esteem—have been met, you should still "expect that a new discontent and restlessness will soon develop, unless the individual is doing what he is fitted for. A musician must make music, an artist must paint, a poet must write, if he is to be ultimately happy. What a man *can* be, he *must* be" (Maslow, 1954, p. 46).

This is why, in their landmark book *Built to Last*, Jim Collins and Jerry I. Porras say that the most successful, most "visionary" companies inevitably have "almost cult-like" cultures— not because they prize blind obedience to some charismatic leader or preach some weird religious sermon about the end of the world, but because everybody in a visionary culture is a little bit weird in the same way (1994, p. 9). A strong culture doesn't set out to alienate anyone, but it doesn't worry too much about it, either. "If you can't embrace the idea of 'wholesomeness' and 'magic' and 'Pixie dust,'" and if you aren't okay with the idea of hordes of sticky little

Blessed is he who has found his work; let him ask no other blessedness. He has a work, a life-purpose; he has found it, and will follow it!

–Thomas Carlyle,
Past and Present

children running amok, "then you'd probably hate working at Disneyland" (Collins & Porras, 1994, p. 9). In some cases, the contours of a culture become so deeply embedded in the minds of employees that they adopt it, consciously or unconsciously, as an integral part of their identity (Sinek, 2014). Trying to imagine being something else is like trying to imagine having gills instead of lungs.

A unique culture can instill in its employees a feeling of belonging that, at its best, becomes a vocation, a calling, a sense that you have found your proper place in the world. Occasionally, a culture "will fit certain people like a custom-made glove," as Amazon CEO Jeff Bezos wrote in his 2016 letter to shareholders. Of course, more than a few critics have looked upon Amazon's corporate culture with suspicion and sometimes disdain. To these people, Bezos just shrugs: "We never claim that our approach is the right one—just that it's ours—and over the last two decades, we've collected a large group of like-minded people. Folks who find our approach energizing and meaningful."

Chances are, if you're not a good fit for a strong culture, you will "flounder, feel miserable and out-of-place, and eventually leave—ejected like a virus" (Collins & Porras, 1994, p. 9).

The leadership team at Midland Health has implemented a wide variety of measures to encourage a high level of engagement with the culture of ownership. There is a separate Culture of Ownership page on the website that includes the 21-module video course on The Self Empowerment Pledge made available to all employees and their family members (for details, see www.PledgePower.com). At MMH, each day's promise is repeated in the Daily Leadership Huddle in the main lobby. In staff huddles around the hospital, you can see employees participating in reciting the daily promise in groups where most of them don't have to read the promise, because they know it by heart. Most employees have received a set of seven wristbands (one for each of the daily promises) and can be seen wearing them in the hallways. They are also available in the auxiliary gift shop in return for a donation of any size to the employee assistance fund.

Every morning at 8:16 sharp, leaders from all departments gather in the main lobby of the hospital for the Daily Leadership Huddle. As a group, they recite The Pickle Pledge and that day's promise from The Self Empowerment Pledge, and then cover key safety and operational highlights. The meeting lasts exactly 14 minutes. When it is over, a summary is sent electronically to every manager and supervisor for daily unit huddles, where the process is repeated throughout the hospital. Therese Hudson Thrall (2016) titled her article on MMH's leadership huddles, simply and accurately, "How to Improve Hospital Operations and Patient Safety in 14 Minutes a Day."

Many MMH managers have taken their own approach to promoting engagement. The manager of the maternity and newborn unit hired a professional artist to decorate the long hallway of her unit with each of the seven promises of The Self Empowerment Pledge. The Medical Staff Services Department starts each day with The Pickle Pledge and the daily promise, but if someone begins to struggle with negative emotions or feel overwhelmed by the pressures of work, they can call a CODE PICKLE: The code is announced in the hallway, and everyone drops whatever they are doing to gather and, once more, recite The Pickle Pledge as a group. As the individual who came up with the idea put it, "It allows us to regroup and remember who we are, and that we as a team stand behind The Pickle Pledge."

One of the most important mechanisms to inspire a high level of engagement by members of the management team is the Midland Health Leadership Team Pledge that Bob created. (See the sidebar.) Every manager is expected to sign this pledge and live up to its terms.

Midland Health Leadership Team Pledge

As a leadership team at Midland Health, we are committed to building and maintaining a positive workplace environment delivering exceptional care and experiences to our patients and their families. As such, I will:

- Embrace the culture of ownership by modeling the way myself.

- Lead with freedom, democracy, and collegiality, not tolerating fear, control, or intimidation from myself or others.

- Commit to a culture of safety, reducing preventable harm at Midland Health. If anyone mentions the words concerned, uncomfortable, or safety (CUS) in a message, I will make this a priority of mine to resolve immediately.

- Reflect a positive attitude and not complain, but engage in solutions without assigning blame. I choose to work here.

- Be professional in all of my interactions, including:

  - Starting meetings on time

  - Communicating professionally

  - Being present and engaged in the moment: Unplug in meetings (no cellphones, computers, or other distractions) as much as possible.

- Participate in the "Sacred 60" leadership rounding daily from 10:00 to 11:00 am. There should be no meetings, phone calls, emails, text messages, or other distractions during this time except when necessary.

- Engage in professional governance and care innovation and transformation processes to build a more positive workplace environment.

- Assume that everyone is doing their best with the tools they have. I will seek first to understand and then to be understood, setting clearer expectations when needed.

- Consider the following meeting strategies (exceptions for necessary, urgent, or emergent needs):

  - Meeting Purpose. Clearly articulate the purpose of meetings. Challenge frequency, other ways of getting the work done while assuring we are advancing our mission, vision and core values.

  - No Meeting Fridays. This allows for catch up on administrative tasks and plan for the next week.

  - Meeting Respite. No meetings scheduled the full month of July and the last half of December (12-15 to 12-31).

- Build and maintain strong, lasting relationships with our patients, families and the people of our community as an ambassador of Midland Health.

- Hold myself accountable to the highest standards of excellence and to lifelong learning. Earn the respect and trust of our patients, their families, medical staff, colleagues, and the community.

- Work hard. There are no tasks too small to meet Midland Health's mission, vision, and core values.

- Balance my work life (career and ambition) and personal life (health, pleasure, leisure, family, and spiritual development or meditation).

- Recognize, reward, and celebrate the accomplishments of others.

Summary

In a culture of ownership, people are emotionally positive, they are self-empowered, and they are fully engaged. The first step to promoting such a culture is raising the level of intolerance for toxic emotional negativity, as reflected in chronic complaining and gossiping. The Pickle Pledge and The Pickle Challenge for Charity are powerful tools for promoting a more positive emotional workplace. The seven promises of The Self Empowerment Pledge help to promote a spirit of initiative within the organization. The Midland Health Leadership Pledge is a tool for fostering a more highly engaged workforce through leadership example.

Chapter Questions

- How many employees in your organization would sign The Florence Challenge Certificate of Commitment and then make a wholehearted commitment to honor the promise?

- Do your employees believe coworkers reflect positive attitudes, treat people with respect, and refrain from complaining, gossiping, or pointing fingers?

- What charity would you select for donations for The Pickle Challenge for Charity? And would the challenge be greeted with enthusiasm or with a surly rolling of the eyes by your employees?

- Do employees of your organization take responsibility (Monday's Promise of The Self Empowerment Pledge) for their actions and hold themselves accountable (Tuesday's Promise) for their outcomes, or do they make excuses and seek to blame others?

- How many of the managers in your organization would enthusiastically sign a leadership pledge and commit to making the personal and professional changes necessary to truly reflect those promises in their leadership styles?

References

Allnurses. (2014). What do you think is the MOST difficult clinical skill to acquire in your experience? Allnurses forum. Retrieved from http://allnurses.com/general-nursing-discussion/what-do-you-57082.html

American Nurses Association. (2011). Health & safety survey: Hazards of the RN work environment. Retrieved from http://nursingworld.org/FunctionalMenuCategories/MediaResources/MediaBackgrounders/The-Nurse-Work-Environment-2011-Health-Safety-Survey.pdf

Begley, S. (2004, November). Scans of monks' brains show meditation alters structure, functioning. *The Wall Street Journal*. Retrieved from http://www.wsj.com/articles/SB109959818932165108

Bezos, J. (2016). To our shareholders. Amazon. Retrieved from https://www.sec.gov/Archives/edgar/data/1018724/000119312516530910/d168744dex991.html

Doidge, N. (2007). *The brain that changes itself: Stories of personal triumph from the frontiers of brain science*. New York, NY: Viking.

Duhigg, C. (2012). *The power of habit: Why we do what we do in life and business*. New York, NY: Random House.

Feeley, D., & Swensen, S. J. (2016). Restoring joy in work for the healthcare workforce. *Healthcare Executive, 31*(5), 70–71.

Ford, S. (2014). Stress levels at work making nurses ill, survey finds. *Nursing Times*. Retrieved from https://www.nursingtimes.net/exclusive-stress-levels-at-work-making-nurses-ill-finds-survey/5077537.article

Goleman, D. (1995). *Emotional intelligence*. New York, NY: Bantam Books.

Khazan, O. (2016). Can three words turn anxiety into success? *The Atlantic*. Retrieved from http://www.theatlantic.com/health/archive/2016/03/can-three-words-turn-anxiety-into-success/474909

Kraft, T. L., & Pressman, S. D. (2012). Grin and bear it! Smiling facilitates stress recovery. *Psychological Science, 23*(11), 1372–1378.

Landes, D. (2000). Culture makes all the difference. In L. E. Harrison and S. P. Huntington (Eds.), *Culture matters: How values shape human progress*. New York, NY: Basic Books.

Lyubomirsky, S., King, L., & Diener, E. (2005). The benefits of frequent positive affect: Does happiness lead to success? *Psychological Bulletin, 131*(6), 803–855.

Mann, T., Tomiyama, A. J., Westling, E., Lew, A. M., Samuels, B., & Chatman, J. (2007). Medicare's search for effective obesity treatments: Diets are not the answer. *American Psychologist, 62*(3), 220–233.

Maslow, A. H. (1954). *Motivation and personality*. New York, NY: Harper & Row.

Poirot, C. (2016, January 13). Cee-eye-eee-eye-ohh: Farmer at heart Robert Earley cultivates a culture of caring and competence at Tarrant County's public-supported health care system. *Fort Worth Business*. Retrieved from http://www.fortworthbusiness.com/news/health_care/cee-eye-eee-eye-ohh-farmer-at-heart-robert-earley/article_5844814a-ba32-11e5-b142-93872d228bac.html

Pressfield, S. (2012). *The war of art: Break through the blocks and win your inner creative battles*. New York, NY: Black Irish Entertainment.

Schwartz, J., & Begley, S. (2002). *The mind and the brain: Neuroplasticity and the power of mental force*. New York, NY: Regan Books.

Sinek, S. (2014). *Leaders eat last: Why some teams pull together and others don't.* New York, NY: Portfolio/Penguin.

Stillman, J. (2016). Gratitude physically changes your brain, new study says. *Inc.* Retrieved from http://www.inc.com/jessica-stillman/the-amazing-way-gratitude-rewires-your-brain-for-happiness.html

Sutton, R. I. (2010). *The no asshole rule: Building a civilized workplace and surviving in one that isn't.* New York, NY: Business Plus.

Tavris, C., & Aronson, E. (2007). *Mistakes were made (but not by me): Why we justify foolish beliefs, bad decisions, and hurtful acts.* Orlando, FL: Harcourt.

Thrall, T. H. (2016). How to improve hospital operations and patient safety in 14 minutes a day. *Hospital & Health Networks.* Retrieved from http://www.hhnmag.com/articles/7036-how-to-improve-hospital-operations-and-patient-safety-in---minutes-a-day

Tugade, M. M., & Fredrickson, B. L. (2004). Resilient individuals use positive emotions to bounce back from negative emotional experience. *Journal of Personal and Social Psychology, 86*(2), 320–333.

Tye, J., & Schwab, D. (2015). *The Florence prescription: From accountability to ownership.* Solon, IA: Values Coach Inc.

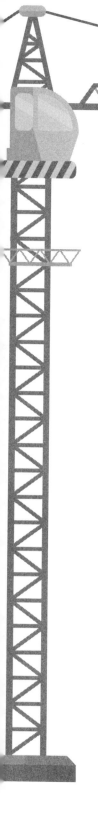

"

If people could understand their core values, they would save years of doubt, confusion, and misplaced energy as they try to find direction for their lives.

"

−Laurie Beth Jones, *Jesus CEO*

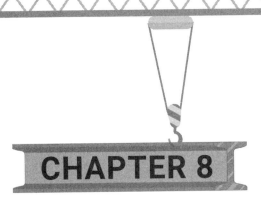

CHAPTER 8

Personal Values and Organizational Values

Chapter Goals

- Explain why healthcare leaders should help employees better understand and act upon their personal values.

- Describe the Values Coach course on The Twelve Core Action Values, which has played a vital role in the cultural transformation at Midland Health.

- Discuss the importance of fostering coherence between the personal values of individual employees and the stated core values of the organization, because while organizational values define strategy, personal values shape culture.

At the beginning of this book, we said that culture does not change unless and until people change; that people will not change unless they are given new tools and structure and the inspiration to use them; and that people will not sustain new attitudes, behaviors, and habits unless those are coherent with their own, underlying personal values. Perhaps paradoxically, the most significant impact of the Culture of Ownership initiative at Midland Health has come not from the work that has been done on culture, but rather from helping people think about, and act upon, their own personal values. The Twelve Core Action Values is a comprehensive and systematic course on values-based life and leadership skills. At Midland Health and other participating organizations, the course is taught by employees who have become Certified Values Coach Trainers (CVCT). They in turn share the course with coworkers, typically in a 2-day class format.

Most people intuitively have good values and generally try their best to live those values. But it is the rare individual who has actually defined those values with any level of specificity, much less adopted a disciplined practice of monitoring how those values are reflected in the decisions they make and in the actions they take. Because they have not clearly defined their personal values, there's often a disparity between the values they reflect in the workplace and the values they reflect at home. As one example, it's hard to imagine that a nurse who bullies others on the unit would behave in the same way with children at home (at least we hope not!).

Paradoxically, one of the most effective ways to inspire employees to embrace the core values of the organization is to use a formal structured process to help them crystallize and actualize their own personal values. Here are five reasons it makes sense for an organization to conduct classes on values-based life and leadership skills for employees.

Overcome Performance Barriers: The collective self-image and self-talk of your employees creates an invisible ceiling on the performance potential of your organization. Thinking about, and acting upon, one's deepest personal values is a sure way of confronting the toxic voice of self-talk and overcoming inner barriers that prevent people from doing their best, giving their best, and being their best.

Enhance Commitment and Loyalty: Roger Herman (*Impending Crisis: Too Many Jobs, Too Few People*) documented an almost direct relationship between the strength and seriousness of an organization's values and its turnover rate. Considering the high cost of turnover, investing in values training can have a substantial long-term payback.

Establish Behavioral Expectations: It is much easier to enforce behavioral expectations when employees see transgressions such as gossiping, bullying, and other forms of toxic emotional negativity for what they really are: violations of personal values. Acting on personal values is the difference between performing because your feet are being held to the fire (accountability) and performing because you are inspired by a fire within (ownership).

Promote Employee Health and Fitness: Participants in the Culture of Ownership courses quit smoking, lose weight, and commit to fitness regimens when they are (finally) doing it because they're motivated by personal values rather than by worries about the opinions of other people.

Enhance Risk Management: Virtually every catastrophic failure of business ethics is at its root a failure of personal values. When a hospital is charged with the inappropriate implementation of cardiac stents, for example, it often reflects a failure on the part of the procedure room team to confront cardiologists who put their personal financial interest ahead of patients' interests.

About The Twelve Core Action Values Course

The Values Coach course on The Twelve Core Action Values is a 60-module curriculum on values-based life and leadership skills. The values featured in The Twelve Core Action Values course are universal and eternal, regardless of an individual's political opinions, religious belief or nonbelief, ethnic background, or any other factor: From Authenticity to Leadership, these are the values everyone can aspire to.

Each of the 12 values is reinforced by four cornerstones, which in turn include practical action strategies for making that value a bigger part of one's life. This is the way the course is structured:

- **The Twelve Core Action Values:** These are the values that structure the course. The first six values (Authenticity, Integrity, Awareness, Courage, Perseverance, and Faith; see Figure 8.1) build a solid foundation of character strength. The second six values (Purpose, Vision, Focus, Enthusiasm, Service, and Leadership; see Figure 8.2) are the fuel for effective action and for making a difference in the world.

- **The 48 Cornerstones:** Each value includes four cornerstones. These are the building blocks by which values become real, the criteria by which someone answers the question "How do I know that I am living my values?"

- **Action Strategies:** Without action, values are little more than good intentions. The Twelve Core Action Values curriculum includes innovative and effective strategies for helping people achieve their most authentic dreams by living in harmony with their deepest values.

In the context of this course, values are more than high-minded aphorisms that often grace success posters—they are skills that can be learned and practiced. We have nothing against success posters (in fact we love them), but living one's values, as opposed to talking about them, is hard work.

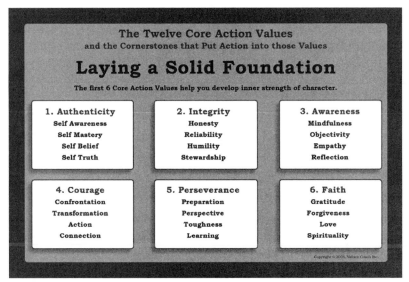

Figure 8.1 *The first six values of The Twelve Core Action Values course.*

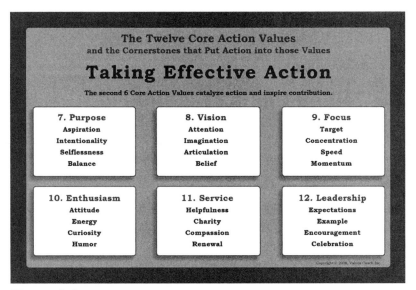

Figure 8.2 *The second six values of The Twelve Core Action Values course.*

For example, Core Action Value #1 is Authenticity. The first cornerstone of authenticity is self-awareness. And one of the best ways to enhance self-awareness is to write in a journal, so the Values Trainer website includes a downloadable, 360-day journal covering 1 of the 12 values and its four cornerstones for each month. For the Midland Year of Values project, Midland Health created a 12-month calendar with each month focused on one of The Twelve Core Action Values to inspire participants to think about how they can be more authentically guided by their values every month of the year.

In the second year of the Values and Culture initiative at Midland Health, 40 individuals participated in a 5-day workshop to become Certified Values Coach Trainers. A second cohort of 20 Values Trainers was recruited the following year. This eclectic group included staff and supervisors from nursing, food service, environmental services, and many other departments. New employees all take the course, and it is now offered to medical staff members and their office employees.

The structure of the course reflects the culture of ownership philosophy. Values Trainers are immersed in the content and given extensive resources for teaching the course, but they are not given a script to follow. Quite to the contrary, they are encouraged to take ownership for the course and teach it in a way that allows them to use their strengths in the best way. Furthermore, because Values Trainers team-teach the course in groups of two, three, or four, they are able to capitalize on the strengths of each member of that team. Over time, as a result of the sharing of ideas between teams, the classes as taught by these teams have become more similar as they have adopted approaches that have been proven to work best, though the classes are still far from identical.

It is, of course, impossible to fully cover personal values in just 2, or even 5, days. Any one of the 12 values, or of the 48 cornerstones that underpin those values, could be covered in a full-semester college course. This course is intended to spark personal reflection and rededication to values on the part of participants.

People take different lessons from the class, depending on who they are, what they do, and where they are in life. The post-course evaluation question "What is the most important thing you got from this course?" can have as many different responses as there were participants in that session.

Results of The Twelve Core Action Values Course

We have heard many stories from course participants about how The Twelve Core Action Values course has changed their lives—stories from people who have reduced or eliminated financial debt, quit smoking, applied for or completed graduate school, changed their approach to parenting, started working on long-postponed books that they'd always said they would write someday, and many others. One new employee, who came to work in the MMH Facilities Department after having been laid off from his job of many years in the oil fields, told Bob that the course gave him a completely different perspective on what work life could and should be. He said that while he'd initially applied to work at MMH just to make ends meet, he now hoped to stay there the rest of his career.

One of the questions that participants face when learning about Core Action Value #1 (Authenticity) is this: What would you do if every job paid the same and had the same social status? Leah knew instantly that her answer to this question was that she would be a writer—but that was not her job at the time. After completing the course, she approached her manager and asked about the possibilities of starting a writing career at MMH. Today, Leah is a writer, working on projects as diverse as public relations documents and the hospital's Magnet® application. She has also become one of MMH's 60 Values Trainers.

There have been frequent occasions where class participants who are overtly skeptical on Day 1 become enthusiastic
participants during Day 2—in fact, several such individuals have become Values Trainers themselves. But someone
who is so overtly negative as to disrupt the class must be
pulled aside during a break and given the choice of changing his attitude (or at least appearing to do so) or being asked
to leave. The latter option has happened only once or twice.
Unfortunately, there are (increasingly rare) occasions when
one or two toxically cynical employees threaten to ruin the
experience for everyone else.

Core Action Value #1: Authenticity

The greatest triumph of the human spirit is to successfully
become the person you were meant to be; the greatest tragedy is to successfully pretend to be someone else because you
think the pay or the status will be higher. Achieving authenticity is a process, not an outcome; "meant to be" does not
necessarily mean easy, inevitable, or preordained. You're
more likely to achieve authenticity by building on your few
greatest strengths than by trying to compensate for your many
weaknesses. This value is the ultimate source of personal
motivation—after all, who wants to be a phony? The
cornerstones of authenticity are self-awareness, self-mastery,
self-belief, and self-truth.

Values Clarity Changes Lives

When Fillmore County Hospital CEO Paul Utemark says
that, as a result of the hospital's work for a culture of ownership, "I got a whole new team and didn't have to change the
people, because they changed themselves," he means it at
the family level as well as at the organizational level. When

Utemark's son Derek completed the course on The Twelve Core Action Values, he was employed as a driver for hospital vehicles, but he wasn't happy. His answer to the question he was asked for Core Action Value #1 (Authenticity)—"What would you do if every job paid the same and had the same social status?"—was not "Driving a truck." It was "Law enforcement." He went back to school and now works as a deputy sheriff in Thurston County, Nebraska. He enjoys serving the people and has learned a lot in his new role, especially about himself.

Core Action Value #2: Integrity

The saying "If you know who you are, then you will always know what to do" forms a bridge between authenticity and integrity. The root of the word *integrity* is *integer*, which has both an inner and an outer dimension. It means that you can be relied on to be consistent at home and at work, and that, as Mother Teresa said, you appreciate that we are all children of the same God. Trust, respect, and reputation are not values— they are attributes that are earned by being a person of integrity. The cornerstones of integrity are honesty, reliability, humility, and stewardship.

Core Action Value #3: Awareness

In *Notes on Nursing* (1860), Florence Nightingale said that the ability to acutely observe is more important than compassion or clinical skills in determining quality patient care. Awareness is the essential ingredient of employee engagement and the antidote to most medical mishaps caused by disengagement and carelessness. Awareness is also a fundamental ingredient of emotional intelligence and personal happiness. It has both an inner and outer dimension; a spatial and a temporal dimension. Awareness is the key to success in virtually every dimension of life—as a parent, caregiver, manager, salesperson, and as a time and money manager. The cornerstones of aware-ness are mindfulness, objectivity, empathy, and reflection.

Core Action Value #4: Courage

Fear is a reaction; courage is a decision. Fear is the emo-tion that people feel when they do brave things. Especially in today's uncertain world, it is essential to teach people practi-cal skills for living with courage in an age of anxiety. No fear, no courage; big fear, big courage. Distinguish among anxiety, fear, and worry, and understand why it's important to proper-ly diagnose each emotional state. The cornerstones of courage are confrontation, transformation, action, and connection.

Core Action Value #5: Perseverance

Fear is a reaction, courage is a decision, and perseverance is making that "courage decision" every day. Each of the seven promises of The Self Empowerment Pledge help to fortify the commitment to persevere. Every great accomplishment was once the "impossible dream" of a dreamer who refused to quit in the face of adversity. And the bigger the dream, the greater will be the challenge. Obstacles and setbacks are not optional—they are an inevitable part of the journey. The cor-nerstones of perseverance are preparation, perspective, tough-ness, and learning.

Core Action Value #6: Faith

Faith as a value is not about religion—*everyone* needs faith. Faith is the marriage of fidelity—being faithful to a person, an organization, a cause—and trust—having faith in a person, an organization, a cause. The Four Pillars of Faith are faith in yourself, faith in other people, faith in the future, and faith in something beyond the visible material world (or what some people call a Higher Power and some call God). Faith in yourself is essential to personal and professional accomplishment; faith in other people is essential to bringing down silo walls; and faith in the future inspires you through the difficult times of today. Faith as a value is reflected in genuine acceptance, as opposed to mere tolerance, of every other human being. The cornerstones of faith are gratitude, forgiveness, love, and spirituality.

Core Action Value #7: Purpose

Here's the first line of Rick Warren's book *The Purpose Driven Life*: "It's not about you" (2002, p. 3). A purpose is broader than a mission; purpose is lifelong and never "mission accomplished." The work you choose to do and the attitude with which you choose to do that work are the hammer and chisel with which you carve the statue of "you." The choices you make determine whether that statue becomes the authentic best self or something lesser. The cornerstones of purpose are aspiration, intentionality, selflessness, and balance.

Core Action Value #8: Vision

Vision is the art of seeing what is invisible to others (Jonathan Swift), and it is a gift that only humans seem to have. With vision as a personal value, you can remember the future more clearly and more accurately than you can remember the past. Visualization and vision work together; visualization is seeing the process, and vision is seeing the outcome; visualization is the verb, and vision is the noun. The cornerstones of vision are attention, imagination, articulation, and belief.

Core Action Value #9: Focus

As you clarify your purpose and your vision, you must be willing to focus your time, energy, relationships, and material resources on achieving that purpose and fulfilling that vision. How you spend your time and money says more about what your values are than what you say they are. According to the Pareto principle (known as "the 80–20 rule"), about 20% of your effort creates 80% of your results; you create leverage by spending less time on trivia and other people's priorities and more time on your most important goals. Focus is the essential discipline of transforming the vision of tomorrow into the reality of today. It is a particular challenge in today's attention-deprived world, which makes it all the more important that leaders teach people the required skills. A blending of focus and enthusiasm (see the following section) constitutes a left-brain, right-brain formula for enhanced productivity. The cornerstones of focus are target, concentration, speed, and momentum.

Core Action Value #10: Enthusiasm

Enthusiasm is a master value in that being enthusiastic makes it easier to live all of the other values, while a lack of enthusiasm makes it harder. As Ralph Waldo Emerson said, nothing great was ever achieved without enthusiasm. To be enthusiastic, you must eliminate toxic emotional negativity, stoke positive emotions, and work to be cheerful and optimistic. Enthusiasm is the catalyst for creating self-fulfilling prophecies and memories of the future. Without enthusiasm, you won't make the commitment, do the work, and recruit the help you need to achieve your most important goals. An organization filled with enthusiastic spark plugs will beat one staffed with disengaged zombies every time. (The Pickle Pledge and The Pickle Challenge for Charity are great tools to spark both personal and organizational enthusiasm; see Chapter 7). The cornerstones of enthusiasm are attitude, energy, curiosity, and humor.

Core Action Value #11: Service

Service is an outer reflection of you as your best self, and of the other 11 Core Action Values—to paraphrase Kahlil Gibran, service is love made visible. Service is what you do for others, and it's the attitude with which you do it. It is Thursday's Promise of The Self Empowerment Pledge in action (see Chapter 7). Service to others is the surest way to escape the trap of the iron triangle of false personality (ego, emotion, ambition). Here's a law of the universe: Whatever you most need in life, the best way for you to get it is to help someone else get it who needs it even more than you do. The cornerstones of service are helpfulness, charity, compassion, and renewal.

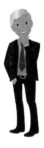

A Note from Joe

I was asked to speak at a conference of operating room managers, the theme of which was "It's Not Florence's OR Anymore." While I agreed with the central theme with regard to the physical dimensions of facilities, technologies, and technical skills, I argued that when it comes to a commitment to compassionate service, most hospitals need to be more, not less, like Florence Nightingale's Scutari Barrack Hospital. ■

Core Action Value #12: Leadership

Anyone who makes a good-faith effort to practice Core Action Values through 1–11 will become the sort of person who, leading by example, influences and inspires others. And that is an excellent definition of what it means to be a leader. Management is a job description; leadership is a life decision. You don't need a management title to be a leader, and in today's turbulent world, leaders are needed in every corner, not just in the corner office. "Proceed until apprehended" isn't just an antidote to learned helplessness—it's also a great formula for a leadership mindset. Transactional leadership is running the business; transformational leadership is changing people—helping others be their best selves and achieve their most important goals in life. Leadership inspires loyalty, and loyalty is to the organization (and the family) what gravity is to the solar system. The cornerstones of leadership are expectations, example, encouragement, and celebration.

Fostering Values Coherence

When teaching the course on The Twelve Core Action Values, Certified Values Coach Trainers (CVCT) challenge course participants to make the connection between those personal values and the core values of the organization. Here are examples, one for each value:

- Core Action Value #1, Authenticity: How does the self-awareness cornerstone complement Strengths Finder, Myers Briggs, or other personal inventory processes we've used in the past?

- Core Action Value #2, Integrity: How does the stewardship cornerstone help us promote more careful use of our organization's resources?

- Core Action Value #3, Awareness: How can the empathy cornerstone help us promote better communication between departments and minimize the silo effect?

- Core Action Value #4, Courage: How can the connection cornerstone help us do a better job of managing courageous conversations in difficult situations?

- Core Action Value #5, Perseverance: How can the toughness cornerstone help us enhance mental toughness and emotional intelligence to more effectively deal with the inevitable challenges of the healthcare environment?

- Core Action Value #6, Faith: How can the forgiveness cornerstone help us foster a culture where people do not engage in pointing fingers and blaming others?
- Core Action Value #7, Purpose: How can the balance cornerstone help us reduce stress in the workplace?
- Core Action Value #8, Vision: How can the attention cornerstone help us identify out-of-the-box opportunities in the marketplace?
- Core Action Value #9, Focus: How can the concentration cornerstone help us not waste time and emotional energy on unproductive activities?
- Core Action Value #10, Enthusiasm: How can we use the curiosity cornerstone to encourage employees to seek great ideas outside of work?
- Core Action Value #11, Service: How can the compassion cornerstone help us be more nonjudgmental toward patients and coworkers?
- Core Action Value #12, Leadership: How can the encouragement cornerstone help us foster a support group mindset in our organization?

This exercise helps to make explicit the linkage between the personal values that shape culture and the organizational values that define strategies.

From Intention to Action

Without action, values are just good intentions, so when teaching the course on The Twelve Core Action Values, CVCTs emphasize practical tools for personal change. One of the most popular is the Direction Deflection Question (DDQ): Will what I am about to say or do help me achieve an important goal and be my best self? This question is infinitely adaptable. Some of the variations adopted by MMH employees include:

- Will what I'm about to put in my mouth help me achieve my goal of losing 25 pounds?

- Will what I'm about to say to my coworker help to build a more positive relationship?

- Will what I'm about to spend the next hour doing help me achieve my goal of earning a Doctor of Nursing Practice degree?

- Will what I'm about to spend my hard-earned cash on help me achieve my goal of being debt-free within 2 years?

Practical tools like the DDQ—and The Pickle Pledge and The Self Empowerment Pledge—help people put action into their values, and as they see positive results reinforces their commitment to those values.

Summary

One of the best ways to inspire employees to embrace the core values of an organization is to help them more effectively define and act upon their own personal values. The Twelve Core Action Values is a systematic course on values-based life and leadership skills used by Midland Health and other organizations to help build a culture of ownership on a foundation of values.

Chapter Questions

- Does your recruiting process help you ascertain whether the personal values of job candidates are coherent with the core values of the organization?

- Do your new employee orientation and employee continuing education programs include content that will help people do a better job of clarifying and acting upon their personal values?

- Does your performance appraisal process include provision for assessing how effectively employees reflect both organizational values and personal values in their work?

References

Nightingale, F. (1860). *Notes on nursing: What it is, and what it is not.* New York, NY: D. Appleton.

Warren, R. (2002). *The purpose driven life: What on earth am I here for?* Grand Rapids, MI: Zonderan.

"

Employees today seek to work for a company and leaders with whom they feel proud to be associated and who treat them like active contributors, not passive producers. They want to work for leaders who appreciate the value they add and rely on their passions and talents to every extent possible.

"

–Michael Frisina, *Influential Leadership*

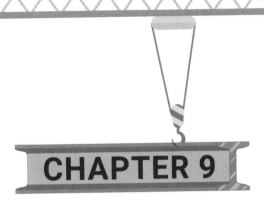

Leadership for a Culture of Ownership

Chapter Goals

- Describe new theories of organizational leadership and distinguish between transactional leadership and transforming leadership.
- Describe the four dimensions of values-based leadership: character, expectations, fellowship, and quest.
- Describe 14 lessons for building a culture of ownership from the experience of Midland Health.

L eadership is one of the most important aspects of any organizational culture. Almost nothing is quite so instrumental in the making or breaking of mission and vision, operations, and strategies. In today's hypercompetitive, turbulent, and uncertain (occasionally terrifyingly uncertain) healthcare environment, one of the most important responsibilities of leadership is to foster leadership at every level of the organization—to promote a culture of ownership.

A purely hierarchical culture is governed like an autocracy. It relies on the industrial/military model of top-down, command-and-control management. Not for nothing does Daniel Goleman, with coauthors Richard Boyatzis and Annie McKee, call this style "commanding" leadership: It consists primarily of issuing commands (and making sure they are obeyed via stern warnings and intimidation) (2013, p. 76). An autocratic organizational structure will spawn a culture that demands subservience ("obey!"), efficiency ("do more with less!"), and specialization ("not my job!"). Behavior is vigilantly supervised; errors are sternly corrected; failure is not tolerated. Power comes from the top, and people do what they're told.

To anyone paying attention, it is increasingly clear that this kind of culture and structure is a poor fit for healthcare organizations. Federal regulations and inspections aren't going away any time soon, of course, nor are standards of practice and accreditation procedures laid down by professional organizations. But the existence of safe, high-quality, low-cost care cannot be ensured by the board, senior management, or select members of the medical staff acting alone. Every chief officer and medical specialist could work 168-hour weeks and it wouldn't be nearly enough. To be a great organization in today's world not only takes a village; the organization must *be* a village where everyone displays a spirit of citizenship and ownership.

Complexity: A Brave New World

Students and scholars of organizational structure often point out that management and leadership are not the same thing. It is often said that "[M]anagers are people who do things right, and leaders are the people who do the right thing" (Bennis & Nanus, 1985, p. 21). Management's basic duty is to keep the machine humming smoothly along: Enforce the rules, organize the staff, delegate tasks, catch mistakes. These tasks are necessary to the smooth functioning of any organization, and they are especially indispensable in healthcare. But always remember that managers are managers solely by virtue of their position on the organizational chart. Some managers are great, profound, powerful leaders. Others function more like bureaucrats who keep the train running on schedule but do little to inspire the passengers.

Fortunately, leadership does not require a management title. Leaders are not born, or promoted into being; they're forged by experience, hardened by discipline, and polished by training and study. Without effort, diligence, and skill, a "born leader" is a waste of potential.

Recent healthcare theory and leadership literature draws heavily on complex adaptive systems (CAS), an interdisciplinary field of study indebted to the mind-bending insights of quantum mechanics, chaos theory, and evolutionary biology. This idea was clearly stated by Margaret Wheatley in *Leadership and the New Science*: "Our concept of the organization is moving away from the mechanistic creations that flourished in the age of bureaucracy. We now speak in earnest of more fluid, organic structures, of boundaryless and seamless organizations. We are beginning to recognize organizations as whole systems, construing them as 'learning organizations' or as 'organic' and noticing that people exhibit self-organizing capacity" (2006, p. 15).

Understanding the networked interconnectedness of patients and health, providers and practice, and even the clinical environment itself will, researchers hope, help practitioners develop the skills they need to cope with, and be effective in, the fast-paced world of modern healthcare: "It is at the edge of chaos that new order emerges and systems evolve while also maintaining their identities" (Crowell, 2010, p. 28).

In a world rife with uncertainty and complexity, health-care practitioners must find new and pragmatic ways to lead, without compromising ethics. This emergent form of egalitarian leadership seeks to overcome the linear, mechanical, hierarchical model of management in favor of dynamic interconnection, interpersonal relationships, and organic adaptation: "Leaders who treat people in the organization as self-organizing and self-renewing and who see the work as being accomplished through relationships are complexity leaders" (Crowell, 2010, p. 30). The current situation demands adaptability, improvisation, and a tolerance for unpredictable events. You should, then, begin to think of "leadership as a collaborative and relational activity that generates high openness and trust, with a shared responsibility, and no longer focuses on one person as 'leader'" (Piggot-Irvine, Henwood, and Tosey, 2014, p. 1). Leadership must become flexible and adaptive, ready to fit shifts in context and surprising circumstances.

Transactional and Transformational Leadership

The conventional definition of leadership—"the ability to influence others"—is not bad as far as it goes, but it's important to note its limitations. The thief who smashes your car window and steals your stereo has a great deal of influence on your life, but it would be silly to call that person a "leader." What if the definition were refined to "the ability to influence others in order to achieve a goal"? Well, then manipulative sociopaths and con artists would be called "leaders," too.

In his Pulitzer Prize-winning book *Leadership* (1978), James MacGregor Burns described two essentially different models of leadership: transactional and transformational.

Transactional leadership

In a transactional leadership model, the leader-follower relationship is structured like an economic exchange: Both parties understand the costs and expectations, and neither gives more than is required. It is a barter system—a day's wages for a day's work, an A+ grade for a perfect score. Of course, transactional leaders can offer incentives (awards, promotions, pay raises, quarterly bonuses) to motivate productivity, or the threat of punishment compliance (insults, probations, pay cuts, public humiliation, threatening job security) to motivate baseline compliance. But both the carrot and the stick are extrinsic motivators.

Such incentives might be sufficient for the factory line or an investment bank, but a healthcare organization is neither, and it should not be run as though it were.

It is perfectly possible for a person to "perform extrinsically motivated actions with resentment, resistance, and disinterest or, alternatively, with an attitude of willingness that reflects an inner acceptance of the value or utility of the task" (Ryan and Deci, 2000, p. 55). But when the motivation to perform is intrinsic to the performer, the task is done for the satisfaction of doing it.

Intrinsic motivation can't be bought or cajoled into existence—it can only be facilitated or undermined. Precisely for this reason, writes Burns (1978, p. 44), "[T]he transformational leader's fundamental act is to induce people to be aware or conscious of what they feel—to feel their true needs so strongly, to define their values so meaningfully, that they can be moved to purposeful action." Pay attention to the phrasing. The leader doesn't move the follower—the leader induces the follower to be moved.

This is why the only true empowerment is self-empowerment: Leaders can do everything in the world to enable their followers, but they will be empowered only when they do the moving themselves. So we would add to the definition: Leaders are people who both *influence* others to do the work and who *inspire* them to take ownership for the work.

Transformational leadership

People won't quit a mission; they will only quit a job.

People won't leave a team; they will only leave an organization.

People won't desert a leader; they will only desert a boss.

—Joe Tye: *All Hands on Deck: 8 Essential Lessons for Building a Culture of Ownership*

Transformational leadership, by definition, changes people—but at its most powerful, it "inspir[es] followers to commit to a shared vision and goals for an organization or unit" (Bass & Riggio, 2006, p. 4). Transforming leaders elevate people to a higher plane of personal values, moral ethics, and performance expectations that are woven into a shared vision. That common vision is the spine of a culture: Purpose creates community; it demands mastery; it self-directs, but does not tolerate indifference.

Transformational leaders are effective in organizations because, instead of taking other employees along for the ride, they allow employees to drive—or, more accurately, they let employees be driven. According to Daniel Pink (2011), the cultures that best facilitate the highest, best form of drive—spontaneous, engaged, joyful work—treasure three things above all:

- **Purpose:** A cause that is bigger than, and allows employees to transcend, egoism and self-interest (the agreed-upon destination)
- **Autonomy:** The ability to work toward goals by making choices (the freedom to find one's own way)
- **Mastery:** The sustained opportunity to develop useful skills and accumulate useful knowledge through engaged, deliberate practice (the journey itself)

Leadership and the Invisible Architecture

One of the most important benefits of being clear about your organization's Invisible Architecture is that it helps you foster leadership at every level. Because leadership "can occur at all levels and by any individual," it is crucial for leaders "to develop leadership in those below them" (Bass & Riggio, 2006, p. 2). Leaders might not be able to "empower" people, but they can—with careful design of the Invisible Architecture—create an environment in which employees empower themselves, in which they are transformed and, through their example, work to transform others in a positive way. This is a culture with a great attitude.

Attitude ultimately means *individual* attitude—the predispositions and emotions that are characteristic of individual people—though there is a thin line between *attitude* and *personality*. Positive-minded people aren't immune to bad moods and bad days, of course, but when a person goes to bed seething, wakes up sneering, and then complains all day, you're dealing with a lousy attitude. Culture is an organization's personality. Every culture has its own predispositions and tendencies. Former Zappos culture strategist Robert Richman (2015, p. 15) takes this idea to its logical conclusion: *"Culture is a feeling"* (italics in original). When you're in a great culture, you immediately know that the leadership isn't just on the 25th floor—it's all around you. And in today's world, leaders are needed in every corner, not just in the corner office.

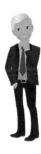

A Note from Joe

The day I visited Antelope Valley Hospital in Lancaster, California, a contentious negotiation with the union representing the hospital's registered nurses had just been concluded, narrowly avoiding a strike. When then-CEO John Rossfeld introduced me to his team, he paraphrased a line that was spoken by a union steward in *The Florence Prescription*: Remember that regardless of our differences, we are all in this together. He encouraged his managers to set aside any hard feelings that might have been engendered during the protracted negotiations and work hard to rebuild relationships that had been strained over the previous year.

A culture of ownership does not mean that there are not differences—sometimes serious differences—of opinion, and occasional conflicts. It means that people work together in a good faith effort to reach the best solution. And that once the solution has been decided upon, everyone works to see that it is effectively implemented, even if it was not the solution they had argued for before the decision was reached. ∎

The Four Dimensions of Values-Based Leadership

There are four essential characteristics of values-based leadership. These qualities apply in every field of leadership, whether it's leading a large organization, a small business, or even a family.

Dimension #1: Character

Character is destiny, said Heraclitus, and nowhere more so than in leadership. Character is forged through commitment to a higher purpose, nurtured by selflessness, and demands total self-honesty. This gradual process requires a lifelong commitment, but the change can be profound and lasting. Mary Kay Ash taught her beauty consultants sales skills and motivated them with dreams of pink Cadillacs, but she also did something more important: She helped her consultants foster personal character strength, something that remains central to the company today. This is one reason that Mary Kay's company has never been embroiled in the sort of controversy that many other companies in the direct-sales field have encountered.

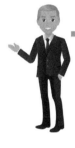

A Note from Bob

The American Organization of Nurse Executives (AONE) is the voice of nursing leadership. As a long-time member and as of this writing president-elect, I have found significant value in belonging to this organization. There are tremendous resources along with the ability to connect with colleagues from around the world. There is value for every nurse, from the student and bedside nurse to the most senior executive. As a leader, I encourage you to be engaged in a professional organization like AONE. ■

Dimension #2: Expectations

You tend to get what you expect. This ancient wisdom has been repeated so often and in so many ways through the ages because it reflects an eternal truth, and nowhere more so than in the relationship between leader and follower. Effective leaders look beyond superficial appearances to find and galvanize hidden strengths in others. A scene early in J. R. R. Tolkien's *The Hobbit* sets the stage for the entire story. Gandalf the Wizard has agreed to help Thorin and his band of dwarves recover the treasure that was stolen from them by a fire-breathing dragon. The dragon has hoarded the treasure deep in a cavern at the bottom of a mountain, and the dwarves need a burglar to sneak in to tell them where the dragon is so that they can recover the treasure without being caught. Gandalf introduces them to Bilbo Baggins, the hobbit. Now, hobbits are short and squat, and they love nothing more than eating, drinking, and sleeping. Thorin, the mighty king of the dwarves, looks down at the little hobbit and sniffs, "Why, he looks more like a grocer than a burglar." Gandalf replies that there's more to Bilbo than meets the eye, that in fact there's more to him than even he sees in himself. The rest of the story is the story of little Bilbo Baggins striving to live up to the expectation created for him by Gandalf the Wizard at the start. By story's end, it is Bilbo who has become the real leader of the group.

Dimension #3: Fellowship

Great organizations tend to be characterized by a strong spirit of fellowship. While fellowship is often in the context of fun with friends, it means much more. It is created when there is common alignment with shared values and a common vision, and a determined commitment to achieving that vision while living those values. A spirit of fellowship is essential to establishing mutual trust in the workplace. Part of the genius of Ray Kroc, founder of McDonald's, was his ability to foster this spirit of fellowship across the company itself, its franchisees, and its suppliers in a unique culture that insiders refer to as McFamily.

Dimension #4: Quest

When Steve Jobs was recruiting John Sculley, then the CEO of Pepsi, to join the executive team at Apple, he asked a question that turned out to be life-changing for Sculley: "Do you want to sell sugar water for the rest of your life or do you want to come with me and change the world?" (Chen, 2011). Creating a spirit of quest, of something bigger than just selling stuff and making money, is the acid test of values-based leadership and of creating a culture of ownership. A quest entails uncertainty and anxiety. (If it were easy and had a guaranteed outcome, it would not be a quest.) Therefore, one of the leader's key responsibilities is helping employees overcome anxiety and channel fear into the energy for constructive action.

Lessons from the Values and Culture Initiative at Midland Memorial Hospital (MMH)

This chapter concludes by sharing the most important lessons we have learned about building a culture of ownership.

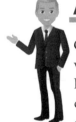

A Note from Bob

Over the past 3 years, MMH has created a new mission, vision, and set of core values. These core values include Pioneer Spirit, Caring Heart, and Healing Mission. One of the cornerstones of Pioneer Spirit is that we will be careful stewards of our resources. As a community hospital, we are facing tough decisions as we complete a cost-transformation exercise over the upcoming 2 years in response to declining reimbursement rates. The cultural transformation we committed to in 2014—embracing a culture of ownership inclusive of The Pickle Pledge, The Self Empowerment Pledge, The Florence Challenge, and The Twelve Core Action Values (provided to all existing employees and now in a 2-day orientation for new employees)—has helped our team better prepare for these and other unforeseen challenges in healthcare. ■

Lesson #1: Assess, don't assume

Research from the University of Iowa Health Management and Policy Department shows that the higher one falls on the organizational chart, the greater the likelihood of wearing rose-colored glasses when making assumptions about culture. The shocking results from the first-round survey at MMH are not atypical for hospitals and other healthcare organizations. As in medicine, so also with cultural transformation—the first step is accurate diagnosis. The first step toward creating a culture of ownership at MMH was the leadership team's honest assessment of its current Invisible Architecture and acknowledgment that change was essential in order to enhance patient satisfaction, community image, and internal operations.

Lesson #2: Be visible

Senior leadership visibility and commitment are essential. At MMH, members of the executive team are fully committed to the entire culture change process and convey to the people who report to them that their support is also mandatory. As one example, every day, every member of the executive team wears the wristband for that day's promise from The Self Empowerment Pledge, and pickle jars for The Pickle Challenge sit in every executive office. (See Chapter 7 for more on The Self Empowerment Pledge and The Pickle Challenge.)

Lesson #3: Don't allow managers to opt out

Middle-management engagement or non-engagement can make or break a cultural transformation process. Before this initiative began, MMH was characterized by a culture of optionality more than by a culture of ownership. As is the case in many organizations, there were no clearly defined cultural expectations, and people were allowed to "opt out" of expectations with an excuse; as long as they performed the elements of their job description, they could not be held accountable for a negative attitude. Creating a sense of ownership had to begin with members of the middle-management team. Middle-management engagement is the single best predictor of building a successful culture of ownership, while middle-management disengagement is the single best predictor of a culture of optionality.

Lesson #4: Engage the medical staff early on

The medical staff can have a huge influence on culture, for better and for worse. When providers are visibly enthusiastic and supportive of culture change efforts, they have a disproportionately positive impact. When a physician participates in The Pickle Challenge for Charity or wears a daily wristband for The Self Empowerment Pledge, for example, people really notice it. On the other hand, if a physician ridicules such efforts, it can be devastating to people who are making the commitment. Thus, it is essential to engage medical staff leadership as early and as fully as possible. At MMH, the elected chief of the medical staff went through the full course to become a Certified Values Coach Trainer, and the MMH Culture of Ownership web page includes a video in which physicians describe how a culture of ownership benefits their practices and their patients.

Lesson #5: Focus on the personal benefits

Remember that everyone listens to radio station WIIFM—What's In It For Me? Give people practical activities, tools, and techniques that they can use not just in their professional work but also in their personal and family lives. The real power of The Pickle Challenge is not just in the way it can reduce complaining and gossiping in the workplace, but in the way it can help individuals who make the commitment learn to be more positive, cheerful, and optimistic in their own lives—and in the way they can "take the challenge home" and share it with their families.

Lesson #6: HR must play a key role

The human resources department must play a key leadership role. From the beginning, Midland's middle managers were told that they could no longer blame HR for their failures to confront and correct inappropriate attitudes and behaviors. HR has played, and continues to play, a leading role in promoting a positive culture of ownership. One of the first things people see when walking into the HR department at MMH is the INSPIRED Award for Values and Culture Excellence that is prominently displayed on the wall.

Lesson #7: Put it in writing

There should be a manifesto or another written document that not only describes cultural expectations but also inspires employee ownership of those expectations. In the case of MMH, the books *The Florence Prescription* (shared during Hospital Week in 2014) and *Pioneer Spirit, Caring Heart, Healing Mission* (shared during Hospital Week in 2015) have served that purpose. During Hospital Week in 2016, every employee received a copy of Joe's book, *Winning the War with Yourself,* with a special message from Joe relating personal self-mastery to participating in building a great organizational culture.

Lesson #8: Give it the feel of a movement

Culture change should begin to have the feel of a movement—beginning with the growing intolerance of toxic emotional negativity in the workplace. At MMH, we hear stories of toxic employees being confronted by coworkers, and even leaving the organization, because they don't want to embrace the new norm of positive expectations. The analogy of the movement to eradicate toxic cigarette smoke from the workplace environment has been especially helpful in communicating expectations that the MMH workplace will be both physically and emotionally healthy. We say more about this in the next chapter.

Lesson #9: Honor legitimate skepticism but be intolerant to cynical opposition

Embrace the skeptics, marginalize the cynics, and plow through resistance. Skeptics are people who ask tough but legitimate questions (such as "How do we know this will work?" and "Who else has taken this approach and what were their outcomes?"), but they ask those questions in good faith; they are more interested in answers than they are in being obstructive. In our experience, once their questions are answered, skeptics become some of the strongest supporters. Cynics, on the other hand, assume that management is acting in bad faith and do everything in their power to make sure that the effort fails. (Cynics love nothing more than to say, "I told you that wouldn't work.") In our experience, once momentum for culture change starts to build, cynics get on board, stop talking, or, in some cases, decide to leave the organization because they can't stand not being the center of attention at the water cooler (and in some cases are actually "voted off the island" by coworkers who are no longer willing to tolerate toxic emotional negativity in the workplace).

Resistance is inevitable. Depending on the organization, it can range from mild skepticism to caustic cynicism. The management team must not allow resistance to derail the culture change commitment. Otherwise, this becomes just another failed program-of-the-month—validating the chief criticism of the cynics who want it to fail.

Lesson #10: Don't allow toxic negativity to poison the process

Unfortunately, a handful of employees never want to see anything that will make for a more positive and productive culture. These are not employees who are pointing out real and legitimate problems—they are the ones for whom nothing is ever right. Because they are often outspoken and, occasionally, domineering, they can appear to have a disproportionately

large influence. Keep this in mind when reading responses
to open questions in a Culture Assessment Survey (CAS),
because people with an ax to grind are often more likely to
take the time to enter a comment than people who have positive perspectives and enthusiastic attitudes.

Lesson #11: Keep it physically visible

Leaders must demonstrate a real and visible commitment that
the culture change initiative will not be just another program-
of-the-month. At MMH, this commitment is reflected in the
visible architecture itself. The walls of the new Culture of
Ownership training center are decorated with its statement of
values as well as The Twelve Core Action Values, The Pickle
Pledge, the seven promises of The Self Empowerment Pledge,
and a large "proceed until apprehended" banner.

Lesson #12: Initiative coherence

Any time a new program is introduced into an organization, it is important to show employees how it builds upon
the work of previous programs so as to avoid the appearance
of "program-of-the-month syndrome." We call this *initiative
coherence*. It ensures that the organization is optimizing and
sustaining the value of previous work.

Lesson #13: Celebrate and share stories

Author Brené Brown says that stories are data with a soul.
We have often seen some of the most cynical resistors change
their attitudes about joining the culture of ownership commitment after hearing about how coworkers have made
meaningful changes in their lives. It's important to have a
mechanism to collect and share such stories.

Lesson #14: Grow the community

Marcy Madrid, Vice President, Planning & Marketing for Midland Health, is leading the Midland Year of Values. She is engaging area colleges, the Midland Independent School District, city government, local businesses and churches, and other entities in a community-wide program to promote The Twelve Core Action Values. Because the culture of a hospital is a subculture of the culture of the community at-large, and because each individual employee goes home to the micro-culture of a family, expanding the commitment gives added momentum to the culture of ownership for the organization.

Lesson #15: Remember the journey never ends

At Values Coach, we often hear the term *program-of-the-month*, but over the years we have learned that whether something is just another program-of-the-month or has a lasting influence on the organization has much less to do with the program than it does with leadership commitment to sustaining the effort until the "program" has become part of that organization's cultural DNA. At MMH, Bob initiated a Daily Leadership Huddle: Every morning at 8:16 sharp, a group assembles in the main lobby for a 14-minute meeting. It begins with someone leading the group in reciting The Pickle Pledge, including the footnote, and that day's promise from The Self Empowerment Pledge. Following that are operational updates. Proceedings are typed and sent to all managers to be shared with all employees.

Every culture change initiative will face a moment of truth (probably more than one) where there is great temptation to give in to the cynics and the naysayers and abandon the quest because it's easier, and often more fun, to move on to an exciting new program than it is to plow through resistance. Refusing to give in at that toughest moment is the quintessential turning point in the hero's journey described by famed mythologist Joseph Campbell.

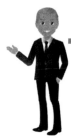

A Note from Bob

At an American Hospital Association's regional policy board meeting, the group had a discussion about community violence and the role that hospitals face in combating violence and addressing its toll on hospital staff. The culture of ownership commitment at MMH, of connecting personal values to our core values, has changed lives and families for the better—so much so that our team is now taking this work to the community in a "Year of Values." We have approached the local community college, school district, and chamber of commerce and the city of Midland. We have created a toolkit for these entities to begin focusing on values as a way to combat teen suicide, bullying, and other violence, as noted on our community health-needs assessment.

Our team is planning to run this as a research project with approval being sought from our Institutional Review Board (IRB) to determine whether this work will have a significant impact on our community's well-being. ■

Summary

Old models of leadership are increasingly counterproductive in today's dynamic healthcare world. Today's leaders must be transforming leaders as well as transactional managers. Values-based leadership requires personal strength of character, high expectations of others, a spirit of fellowship, and imputing a sense of quest to the work.

Chapter Questions

- How would you characterize the leadership styles practiced in your organization?

- Is there a visible commitment to promoting and enforcing the cultural expectations of the organization? What more can be done?

- How does the leadership team assess the culture of the organization? How do they avoid the problem of rose-colored glasses?

- Does the Invisible Architecture of your organization have a seamless connection between the foundation of core values, the superstructure of organizational culture, and the interior finish of workplace attitude, or are there gaps reflected in employees not walking the organization's talk?

References

Bass, B. M., & Riggio, R. E. (2006). *Transformational leadership.* Mahwah, NJ: Lawrence Erlbaum Associates, Inc.

Bennis, W. G., & Nanus, B. (1985). *Leaders: The strategies for taking charge.* New York, NY: Harper & Row.

Burns, J. M. G. (1978). *Leadership.* New York, NY: Harper & Row.

Chen, M. (2011). Scully on Jobs' sugar water legend. *Triangle Business Journal.* Retrieved from http://www.bizjournals.com/triangle/blog/2011/09/scully-on-jobs-sugar-water-legend.html

Crowell, D. M. (2010). *Complexity leadership: Nursing's role in health care delivery.* Philadelphia, PA: F. A. Davis.

Frisina, M. E. (2014). *Influential leadership: Change your behavior, change your organization, change health care.* Chicago, IL: Health Administration Press.

Goleman, D., Boyatzis, R., & McKee, A. (2013). *Primal leadership: Unleashing the power of emotional intelligence.* Boston, MA: Harvard Business Review Press.

Piggot-Irvine, E., Henwood, S., & Tosey, P. (2014). Introduction to leadership. In S. Henwood (Ed.), *Practical leadership in nursing and health care: A multi-professional approach.* Wellington: NZCER, 11–30.

Pink, D. H. (2011). *Drive: The surprising truth about what motivates us.* New York, NY: Riverhead Books.

Richman, R. (2015). The culture blueprint: A guide to building the high-performance workplace. Creative Commons.

Ryan, R. M., & Deci, E. L. (2000). Intrinsic and extrinsic motivations: Classic definitions and new directions. *Contemporary Educational Psychology, 25,* 54–67.

Tolkien, J. R. R. (1966). *The hobbit, or, there and back again.* Boston, MA: Houghton Mifflin.

Wheatley, M. (2006). *Leadership and the new science: Discovering order in a chaotic world.* Oakland, CA: Berrett-Koehler Publishers.

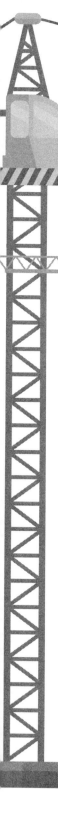

"At the end of the day, just remember that if you get the culture right, most of the other stuff – including building a great brand – will fall into place on its own."

–Tony Hsieh: *Delivering Happiness: A Path to Profits, Passion, and Purpose*

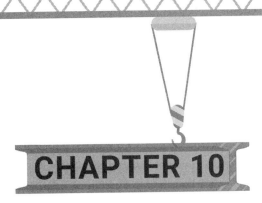

CHAPTER 10

Anatomy of a Change Movement

What the Movement to Ban Public Smoking Has to Teach Healthcare Leaders About Culture Change

In 2005, a CEO named Mike Szymanczyk testified in court that his employer had at one time been "out of alignment with society's expectations of a socially responsible company" (Szymanczyk, 2005, p. 18). The corporation had been subject to public outrage, scandalous lawsuits, and official censure from regulatory officials.

But that all changed, said Szymanczyk, when none other than Mike Szymanczyk himself launched a Corporate Responsibility Task Force to explore how the company could increase its value to society. "Why do we exist?" the task force asked; "What is our positive contribution to society?" (McDaniel & Malone, 2012, p. 1943). From 1997–98, Szymanczyk's team gradually formulated a doctrine of core values that included the following statements:

- "We have the courage to do what's right."
- "As a company, we acknowledge and embrace our role as a responsible, involved citizen and community leader."

These core values, Szymanczyk testified, "mean nothing if they are just words on a card." He said, "They have to be communicated and acted upon" (Szymanczyk, 2005, p. 41). And Szymanczyk was confident that he had been successful in reshaping the organization's identity. True, the company was in the same business, making the same products for the same consumers. But, he said, "It's no exaggeration to say that the culture of this company has been completely transformed over the past eight years" (Szymanczyk, 2005, p. 45). But how did this fundamental transformation take place? What accounted for its success? Ultimately, he said, "[O]ur accomplishments are due primarily to our employees' commitment to the company's mission and values" (Szymanczyk, 2005, p. 223).

Szymanczyk's employer? The Altria Group, better known as Philip Morris, America's largest tobacco company.

The values laid out by Szymanczyk's Corporate Responsibility Task Force have since been wiped from Altria's web presence and replaced by a hodgepodge of tepid corporate slogans ("passion to succeed," "driving creativity into everything we do," "sharing with others") that, if you didn't know any better, have nothing to do with selling Chesterfields or Marlboro Lights. There was not a seamless connection between the noble values of courage and responsibility (the foundation of Invisible Architecture) and a culture that thrives on selling an addictive and deadly product (the superstructure of Invisible Architecture). To prevent cognitive dissonance, something had to change—and for the people at

Altria, it was much easier, and much more profitable, to water down the company's professed values than to try and live them.

One of the most profound cultural changes in the history of the world has been the rapid alteration of perceptions about the acceptability of smoking in public places, and of tobacco companies using television advertising featuring macho cowboys, glamorous (and anorexically thin) women, and cartoon characters to promote a deadly addiction.

When former U.S. Surgeon General Dr. C. Everett Koop called for a smoke-free society in 1986, people wondered what *he* was smoking. Back then, people smoked everywhere: in restaurants, in offices and hospitals, in taxicabs, and even in airplanes. You could hardly escape the ambient stench of cigarette smoke—not even in a hospital. Even in many outdoor locales, such as football stadiums on a Saturday afternoon, a pervasive cloud of cigarette smoke hung in the air. Today, of course, Koop's dream of a smoke-free society has substantially been achieved. From the bars of New York City to the hotel rooms of North Carolina (home of the tobacco industry), smoking has been increasingly relegated to the back of the building, next to the trash bin. Anyone lighting a cigarette on an airplane now would most likely be escorted off the plane in handcuffs. The world has changed dramatically, profoundly, and permanently. It is worth examining how it has happened, because the antismoking movement offers many lessons for the challenge of cultural transformation.

Audacity and the WIIFM Factor

When Millard Fuller founded Habitat for Humanity, his sights were set not on eradicating poverty housing in his hometown of Americus, Georgia, but rather on having "no more shacks" anywhere in the world. But he coupled that audacious goal with a subtle appeal to the people whom he wanted to persuade to donate and to volunteer, because who doesn't wish that they could spend a little time outside, swinging a hammer with friends? Habitat for Humanity was based on a big dream, but it was a dream that appealed to virtually everyone, albeit for different reasons. In 1986, the goal of a smoke-free society was the impossible dream, but it was a dream with a strong WIIFM (What's In It For Me?) factor. Smoking, after all, isn't just unhealthy for those who smoke; it's also unhealthy for nonsmokers upon whom ambient smoke is inflicted. From this perspective, everyone had an incentive to police the policy because all it takes is for one person lighting a cigarette to instantly pollute the lungs of everyone else in the room.

Protect the Lone Nuts

The antismoking movement was started by a small core of what Derek Sivers (2010), in a TED Talk, calls *lone nuts*. These are the movement starters, the people who feel strongly about something and are willing to be labeled as fanatics, as idiosyncratic kooks with an ax to grind. These are the people who galvanize cultural transformation in the organization. They are precious jewels, people whom leadership should treasure and nurture because they have the

> "It is not the law of large numbers or critical mass that creates change, but the presence of a small disturbance that gets into the system and is then amplified through the networks. Once inside the network, this small disturbance circulates and feeds back on itself. As different parts of the system get hold of it, interpret it, and change it, the disturbance grows. Finally, it becomes so amplified that it cannot be ignored."
>
> —Margaret Wheatley, *Leadership and the New Science: Discovering Order in a Chaotic World*

courage to withstand the criticism and ridicule of coworkers in the quest to foster a more positive and productive organization. In a culture change movement, these people are the spark plugs.

Don't Quit Until You Achieve Critical Mass

For many years, the antismoking movement faced fierce resistance and suffered many setbacks. The tobacco industry spent (and continues to spend) hundreds of millions of dollars to fight against any measure that would reduce cigarette sales, while smokers fought for what they claimed to be "smokers' rights" (a term you almost never hear now). It took a while, but eventually the lone nuts began to have an impact. Soon there were no-smoking areas in restaurants, no-smoking rooms in hotels, and smokers were relegated to the back of the airplane (as if that made any difference on cross-country flights). As people began to appreciate these havens of fresh air, demand for them increased gradually at first, and then exponentially. Over time, smokers began to be relegated to the smoking room at the back of the restaurant or the smoking lounge in airports. Then, as a critical mass of people began insisting that they *never* be exposed to toxic cigarette smoke, it was almost as if a cosmic switch had been flipped and the world changed.

The spark plugs in your organization (also known as lone nuts) can be out there on the leading edge for only so long before they burn out, so the leadership challenge is to add "first followers" as quickly as possible so that you achieve a critical mass of participants and the movement becomes self-sustaining. There is quite a bit of research on just where that tipping point of reaching critical mass lies, and it's around 30%. After 30% of the population became intolerant of someone else's cigarette smoke, achieving Koop's vision of a smoke-free society became almost inevitable.

Raise the Bar (but Don't Move the Goalposts)

In the early years of the antismoking movement, people were happy just to have a sanctuary where they could find a respite from the all-pervasive cloud of cigarette smoke that enveloped most buildings. Cigarette advertising, including that which was insidiously designed to induce children into a lifetime of addiction, was so ubiquitous that people hardly noticed it. With each small win—having a designated no-smoking section in restaurants or on airplanes, outlawing cigarette advertising on TV and in movies, banning cigarette vending machines—activists raised the bar and maintained momentum toward the ultimate goal of a world that is free of this perniciously addictive and dangerous product.

The same thing happens with culture change. For example, at Fillmore County Hospital in Geneva, Nebraska, it took a while for employees to realize that CEO Paul Utemark and his team of spark plugs (a.k.a. lone nuts) were serious about eradicating chronic complaining, gossiping, and other forms of toxic emotional negativity from the organization. As people began to appreciate how nice it was to come to work in a more positive emotional environment, they became increasingly less tolerant of coworkers who insisted upon polluting it with whining and rumormongering. Eventually, some of the most negative employees left of their own accord because they simply couldn't stand the fact that nobody wanted to listen to them anymore.

Anyone under the age of 30 can hardly imagine how disgusting it must have been to live and work in a world polluted with toxic cigarette smoke. Talk to a high schooler today about how people used to smoke cigarettes on airplanes, and they are incredulous that an entire society would allow itself to be subjected to that type of chronic poisoning. *They* certainly would never allow the air they breathe, the air their future children will breathe, to be poisoned by someone else's smoke, the way their grandparents unthinkingly did. It is inconceivable to think smoking will ever be tolerated again, but it is also quite certain that the big cigarette companies are always watching for a way to wedge that door open again. Constant vigilance is required to make the change permanent.

As a society, we will never again tolerate, or be forced to endure, toxic cigarette smoke in the workplace. Imagine if the next generation of nurses could say the same thing about toxic emotional negativity—that it simply is not tolerated in organizations that are meant to be places of healing.

References

McDaniel, P. A., & Malone, R. E. (2012, October). The big why: Philip Morris's failed search for corporate social value. *American Journal of Public Health, 102*(10): 1942–1950.

Philip Morris. (2016). How we operate. Retrieved from http://www.pmi.com/eng/about_us/how_we_operate/pages/how_we_operate.aspx

Sivers, D. (2010). Derek Sivers: How to start a movement [video file]. Retrieved from https://www.ted.com/talks/derek_sivers_how_to_start_a_movement

Szymanczyk, M. (2005, April). MES DOJ testimony. Philip Morris Records. Retrieved from https://www.industrydocumentslibrary.ucsf.edu/tobacco/docs/qllm0001

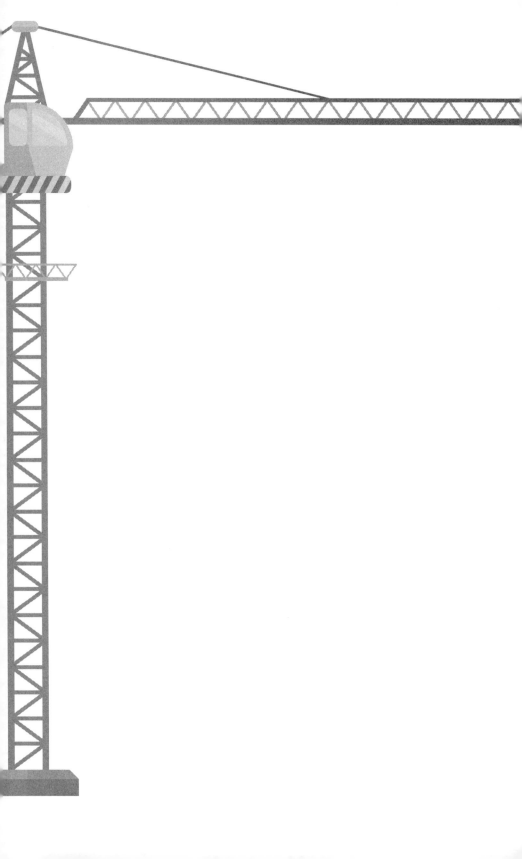

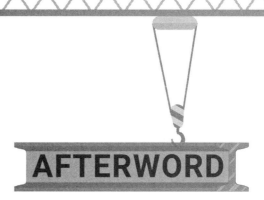

Caring, Ownership, and the Foundations of Excellence

I remember as a new young nurse, steeped in the thrill of graduating nursing school and beginning my professional career, what an exciting moment that was for me. Having had a rather rocky childhood and having not made many good choices up to the moment I chose to be a nurse, this was a celebration greater than simply having graduated. It was a personal triumph for me. Out of this moment grew great expectations that would be demonstrated in my opportunity as a nurse to care, touch people's lives, make a difference in their healing journey, and ultimately in the process, transform my own life.

At the outset, while many of my sentiments and hopes were evidenced in genuine opportunities to care and to serve, I began to notice other feelings emerging out of my experience. Over time, I began to see the real and genuine challenges within my healthcare organization that made it increasingly difficult to authentically express the full capacity of both my competence and care. First and foremost, it did not appear as though the work culture was genuinely oriented to supporting the work I did as a nurse. I found more of my time was spent "working around" a culture and context that was extremely hierarchical, functional, process-oriented, rule-bound, and time-compressed. Ultimately, it appeared that getting work done, checking off boxes, moving patients in-through-out quickly, and doing what was ordered was the true milieu within which the work of nursing was undertaken. Soon, I began to understand some of the cynicism, bitterness, and frank non-engagement I sensed in my more experienced and tenured nursing colleagues and began to sense the same arising in my own nursing spirit. What was especially concerning to me was that the work of nurses comprised at a minimum 50% of the clinical work and resources of the organization, yet the structures and processes of the system did nothing to demonstrate valuing, engaging, investing, and collaborating with one of the health system's most significant caring and clinical resources. In my own mind, this failure was a primordial driver for problems associated with genuine caring, ownership, investment, and engagement, demonstrated by measures of low satisfaction, poor quality, bad attitude, and an environment where genuine caring was the exception rather than the rule. And this frightened me.

Feeling a genuine sense of personal dissonance between my sense of nursing and the work of nursing concerned me enough to want to know more about what drove healthcare systems, decision-making, leadership, and clinical practice. It is this set of questions that has formed the centerpiece of my own clinical and scholarly journey and continues to inform and challenge those efforts some 45 years later. Through this process, the elements of complexity science, adaptive systems, social and relational science, and group psychodynamics have converged to generate a full range of insights that have deepened my understanding of human systems, leadership, and enabling social structures. More than 30 years of comprehensive human dynamics research has yielded some fundamental and strongly validated data that affirms some essential constructs guiding groups, work, and those forces that enable/ disable core human impulses to fully engage lives, relate to others, advance the human community, and affect positive impact going forward.

After these many years in healthcare practice and leadership, I have come to realize that I am not alone in my foundational experiences as a nursing professional and that much of the work of my career has been directed to addressing these original feelings and insights experienced from the very outset of my career. Even after 45 years of clinical and leadership work in healthcare, these concerns remain as valid today (if not more so) as they did when my career began. While much significant progress has been made regarding the science and knowledge affecting adult work structures and behavior, smaller successes have been obtained related to implementation and application in transforming the real world of work. It is because of the set of circumstances that I am most excited by the work of Joe Tye and Bob Dent. Their detailed application of the Invisible Architecture acting as a metaphor for core values, culture, and attitude creates an integral set of dynamics whose interface forms a framework for sustainable ownership and impact.

What we have learned from the past 30 years of human dynamics sciences research is that there is a fundamental interdependence between human group structures, a goodness of fit between strategy and practice, full investment and engagement between the organizational stakeholders, and congruence between the prevailing culture and sustainable behaviors.

Research has shown us that trust is not a driver of meaningful relationships; it is, instead, its product. We know, for example, it is impossible to create sustainable behavioral change unless there is a prevailing infrastructure that is consonant with it and enables it instead of extinguishing it. We know that organizational structure is no more or less important than good work practices and behaviors; indeed, their relationship is symbiotic, and successful organizations cannot operate without the goodness of fit between both.

Leaders, aware of these and other related principles and grounded in human science, must now realize that the work to apply these principles is not sustainable if the overriding organizational effort fails to advance engagement, ownership, and investment. In healthcare, these values drive the triple-aim goals of accelerating levels of patient satisfaction, service excellence, and quality impact, advancing community health and creating a healthy balance in the value equation between the cost of doing business and the price of good business practices. This synthesis articulated by the Invisible Architecture suggested by Tye and Dent is simply not optional in the effort to achieve and to sustain real value. Indeed, it is the challenge of the time. It can easily be said that without the convergence and congruence among structure, culture, values, and ownership, these outcomes can neither be achieved nor sustained.

Looking ahead, the notion of engagement and ownership will need to further represent an increasing understanding of the implications of equity in the balance between an individual's motivation and his or her personal return on investment. Leaders often expect others to invest and to engage in a way that doesn't represent collateral value, inclusivity, and mutuality in decision-making. This negatively affects individuals' lives. As a result, they do not access rewards available to them through demonstrated competence, investment, commitment, and achieving positive value for themselves and the system. This ultimately makes for a very short-term and short-sighted experience for everyone. The organizational landscape is littered with enthusiastic, value-grounded approaches that became incremental merely because they failed to address this delicate yet vital equilibrium.

Finally, ownership is more than just a sense, sentiment, or subset of engagement. Ownership more than implies embracing and investing one's resources and energies. Ownership exemplifies a clear and articulated "quid pro quo" that is palpable and real. It is visualized in organizations that have decisional models where 90% of the decisions are driven by "owners" at the point of service. It is exemplified by the realization that decisions are collateral and that organizational decisions are not exclusively summative (hierarchical) but are instead "distributive." This means substantively that decisional rights are owned by certain people at specific places in the organization simply because they are legitimately there and fulfill Taguchi's requisite: The closer a decision is made to the place where it will be exercised, the lower the cost, the lower the risk, and the higher the sustainability of both the validity and impact of that decision. He indicated that the reverse holds equally true: The further away a decision is made from the place where it will be exercised, the higher the cost, the greater the risk, and the lower the sustainability of its outcome. In short, this means that everyone in an effective system owns particular and identifiable decisions that must be clearly articulated so that they are both understood and rightly exercised. Leaders "allowing" others to make decisions that these people, in truth, need to (or legitimately) own is egregiously paternalistic, creating an infrastructure that does not enable true and sustainable ownership and its essential positive byproducts. However, this mental model is all too frequently apparent in organizations that talk ownership without fully understanding its fundamental characteristics and implications impacting structure, decisions, and behaviors.

All of that said, if the readers of this book look deeply within its contents, all the elements and foundations essential to building a true culture of ownership are evident here.

Accommodating the caveats suggested above, the concerted and consolidated effort around structure, culture, values, and ownership form a durable, 360-degree infrastructure and human dynamic that engages, enthuses, sustains, and enables continuous advancement and growth. The side benefits of this important work are invariably an elevated sense of self-worth, a stronger set of viable and meaningful relationships, a more effective infrastructure for expressing human meaning and advancement, and, not necessarily specific to healthcare but essential to it, a true and palpable caring environment.

This is not to say that this book implies that building and sustaining the frame for organizations that reflect this human dynamic is either easy or quick. Clearly, a century of impeding structures and practices not reflecting these fundamental principles creates a formidable barrier to undertaking this necessary personal, professional, and systemic organizational work. Yet this work is necessary to creating both the formative architecture and behavioral practices that work in concert to enable the resulting caring, value-based human dynamic and its vital positive impact on the health of the human community that drove me and most of my healthcare colleagues to this work in the first place.

Tye and Dent have described an effective algorithm through which this dynamic can unfold, and they provide an effective toolset that is proven to be demonstrably successful. In the final analysis, the reader has only one last lingering question: *What is keeping me from beginning this essential work where I live, lead, and practice?*

–Tim Porter-O'Grady, DM, EdD, APRN, FAAN, FACWS
Senior Partner, TPOG Associates, Inc., Atlanta, Georgia
Professor of Practice, College of Nursing and Health Innovation, Arizona State University, Phoenix, Arizona
Clinical Professor, Leadership Scholar, College of Nursing Ohio State University, Columbus, Ohio, USA
Adjunct Professor, School of Nursing, Emory University, Atlanta, Georgia, USA

INDEX

W

Y

Z

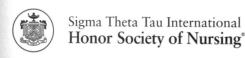
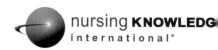

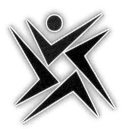

Learn more about how Values Coach can help your organization create a **Cultural Blueprint for your Invisible Architecture**™ of values, culture, and attitude—and build a stronger and more vibrant culture of ownership based on that blueprint. Available services include:

- Working with your leadership team step-by-step through the **cultural transformation process** that culminates with your organization earning the INSPIRED Award for Values and Culture Excellence.

- Producing custom editions of **The Florence Prescription: From Accountability to Ownership** to help you launch The Florence Challenge for a culture that is emotionally positive, self-empowered, and fully engaged.

- Working with your leadership team to launch **The Pickle Challenge for Charity**, including before-and-after administration of the Culture Assessment Survey with a report of observations and recommendations.

- **Leadership retreats**; all-employee assemblies; and special events to inform, inspire, and transform.

- Preparing a team of **Certified Values Coach Trainers** to integrate The Twelve Core Action Values into your organization's cultural DNA.

Values Coach Inc.
Transforming People through the Power of Values
Transforming Organizations through the Power of People

Contact Values Coach at
319-624-3889 or Joe@ValuesCoach.com

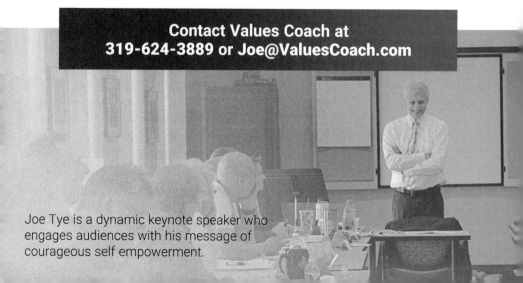

Joe Tye is a dynamic keynote speaker who engages audiences with his message of courageous self empowerment.

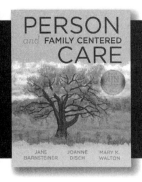 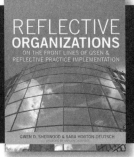 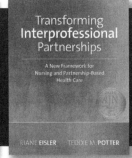 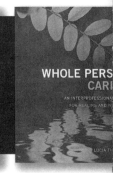

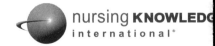

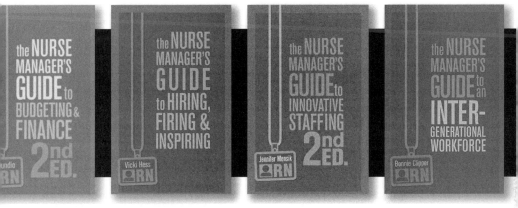
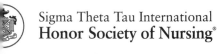
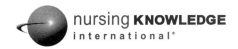

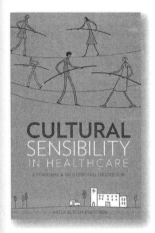
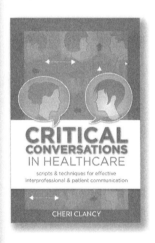
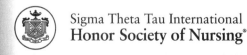
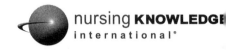

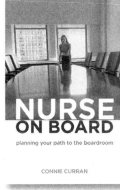
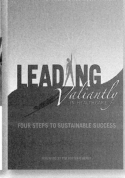
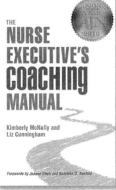
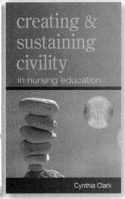

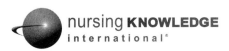

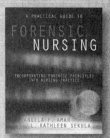
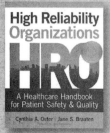
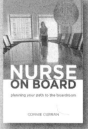
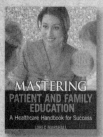
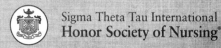
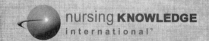